The "I LOVE MY AIR FRYER" Keto Diet

Recipe Book

From *Veggie Frittata* to *Classic Mini Meatloaf*, 175 Fat-Burning Keto Recipes

Sam Dillard of HeyKetoMama.com

Author of *The "I Love My Instant Pot®" Keto Diet Recipe Book*

Adams Media

New York   London   Toronto   Sydney   New Delhi

Thank you to our family and friends for all your support.

To my wonderful husband, Joe—thank you for being my biggest encouragement and making this all possible. There is absolutely no way I could have done this without you.

Joey and Maya, thank you for your patience and being my little taste testers.

This book is for my dad, who for years has always asked, "What's cooking good?" during our Sunday phone calls.

To all my Keto followers, thank you all for your encouragement and support. You all inspire me to be creative every single day.

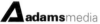

Adams Media
An Imprint of Simon & Schuster, Inc.
57 Littlefield Street
Avon, Massachusetts 02322

First Adams Media trade paperback edition January 2019

ADAMS MEDIA and colophon are trademarks of Simon & Schuster.

For information about special discounts for bulk purchases, please contact Simon & Schuster Special Sales at 1-866-506-1949 or business@ simonandschuster.com.

The Simon & Schuster Speakers Bureau can bring authors to your live event. For more information or to book an event contact the Simon & Schuster Speakers Bureau at 1-866-248-3049 or visit our website at www.simonspeakers.com.

Interior design by Heather McKiel
Photographs by James Stefiuk
Nutritional stats calculated by Melinda Boyd

Manufactured in the United States of America

10 9 8 7 6 5 4 3 2 1

Library of Congress Cataloging-in-Publication Data
Names: Dillard, Sam, author.
Title: The "I love my air fryer" keto diet recipe book / Sam Dillard of HeyKetoMama.com, author of The "I love my instant pot®" keto diet recipe book.
Description: Avon, Massachusetts: Adams Media, 2019. Series: "I love my" series.
Includes index.
Identifiers: LCCN 2018037198 | ISBN 9781507209929 (pb) | ISBN 9781507209936 (ebook)
Subjects: LCSH: Reducing diets--Recipes. | Ketogenic diet. | Hot air frying. | BISAC: COOKING / Health & Healing / Low Carbohydrate. | COOKING / Methods / Special Appliances. | HEALTH & FITNESS / Diets.
Classification: LCC RM222.2 .D5747 2019 | DDC 641.5/63--dc23
LC record available at https://lccn.loc.gov/2018037198

ISBN 978-1-5072-0992-9
ISBN 978-1-5072-0993-6 (ebook)

Contents

Introduction

If you have an air fryer, you already know it's a revolutionary appliance meant to save you time and help you live better. If you still haven't made the leap, you'll be excited to learn just how quickly you'll be hooked and using your air fryer to prepare nearly every meal. But what's so special about air frying?

The air fryer can replace your oven, your microwave, your deep fryer, and your dehydrator and evenly cook delicious meals in a fraction of the time you're used to. If you're looking to provide your family with healthy meals, but don't have a lot of time, the air fryer is a game changer.

An air fryer can also help with your success on the keto diet. One of the many benefits to air frying is the short cooking times it provides. This is especially beneficial when you are hungry and short on time, a recipe for cheating on your diet. Long-term success on a ketogenic diet is often attributed to ease of preparing healthy meals. That's why your air fryer will be your best friend throughout your keto journey and help you stay on track, even on the days when you're short on time.

Throughout this book you'll learn everything you need to know about how and why to use an air fryer as well as some basics that will help you find success following the ketogenic diet. Let's get cooking!

1

Cooking with an Air Fryer

Cooking with an air fryer is as easy as using a microwave. Anybody can do it, and after just a few uses you'll wish you had switched over to this genius method of cooking earlier. This chapter will introduce you to air frying options and maximizing your cooking time and crispness, explain how to keep your air fryer clean, and recommend some accessories that will make your air frying experience even easier and more enjoyable.

While this chapter will cover the basics of using your air fryer, the first step is reading the manual that came with your air fryer. All air fryers are different, and with the recent rise in popularity of the appliance there are a lot of different models on the market. Learning how to use your specific air fryer thoroughly is the key to success and will familiarize you with troubleshooting issues as well as safety functions. Reading over the manual and washing all parts with warm, soapy water before first use will help you feel ready to unleash your culinary finesse!

Why Air Frying?

Air frying is increasingly popular because it allows you to quickly and evenly prepare delicious meals with little oil and little effort. Here are just a few of the reasons you'll want to switch to air frying:

It replaces other cooking appliances. You can use your air fryer in place of your oven, microwave, deep fryer, and dehydrator! In one small device, you can quickly cook up perfect dishes for every meal without sacrificing flavor.

It cooks faster than traditional cooking methods. Air frying works by circulating hot air around the cooking chamber. This results in fast and even cooking, using a fraction of the energy of your oven. Most air fryers can be set to a maximum temperature of 400°F. Because of this, just about anything you can make in an oven, you can make in an air fryer.

It uses little to no cooking oil. A main selling point of air fryers is that you can achieve beautifully cooked foods with little to no cooking oil. While that may be attractive to some because it can mean lower fat content, people following the keto diet can rejoice because it means fewer calories, which still matter if you're doing keto for weight loss.

It has a fast cleanup. With any method of cooking you're sure to dirty your cooker, but with your air fryer's smaller cooking chamber and removable basket, thorough cleanup is a breeze!

Choosing an Air Fryer

When choosing an air fryer, the two most important factors to focus on are size and temperature range. Air fryers are usually measured by quart size and range from about 1.2 quarts to 10 or more quarts. If you're looking to cook meals to feed a family, you might be interested in at least a 5.3-quart fryer that can be used to beautifully roast an entire chicken (see Lemon Thyme Roasted Chicken in Chapter 5), but if you need a small machine because of limited counter space and you're cooking for only one or two, you can definitely crisp up some Jicama Fries (see Chapter 4) with a much smaller air fryer. As for temperature range, some air fryers allow you the ability to dehydrate foods because you can cook them at a very low temperature, say 120°F, for a long period of time (see Beef Jerky in Chapter 3). Depending on the functions you need, you'll want to make sure your air fryer has the appropriate cooking capacity and temperature range.

The Functions of an Air Fryer

Most air fryers are equipped with buttons to help you prepare anything, such as grilling the perfect salmon, roasting an entire chicken, or even baking a chocolate cake.

These buttons are attached to preset times and temperatures based on your specific air fryer. Because of the wide variety of air fryers on the market, all recipes in this book were created using manual times and temperatures. Every air fryer allows you to set these yourself. Still, it is important to know how the cooking programs

work on your air fryer and when to use them.

While some air fryer recipes call for preheating the appliance, this is really more of a personal preference. Some people preheat their air fryers while others just add a few minutes to the cooking time, which is what is done in these recipes. In my personal experience there's no benefit to preheating which is why it is not called for in this book.

Essential Accessories

Your air fryer's cooking chamber is basically just a large, open space for the hot air to circulate. This is a huge advantage because it gives you the option to incorporate several different accessories into your cooking. These accessories broaden the number of recipes you can make in your air fryer and open up options you never would've thought were possible. Here are some of the common accessories.

Metal holder. This circular rack is used to add a second layer to your cooking surface so you can maximize space and cook multiple things at once. This is particularly helpful when you're cooking meat and veggies and don't want to wait for one to finish to get started on the other.

Skewer rack. This is similar to a metal holder, but it has built-in metal skewers that make roasting kebabs a breeze.

Ramekin. Small ramekins are great for making mini cakes and quiches. If they're oven safe, they're safe to use in your air fryer.

Cake pan. You can find specially made cake pans for your air fryer that fit perfectly into the cooking chamber. They also come with a built-in handle so you can easily pull them out when your cakes are done baking.

Cupcake pan. A cupcake pan usually comes with seven mini cups and takes up the entire chamber of your 5.3-quart air fryer. These versatile cups are perfect for muffins, cupcakes, and even egg cups. If you don't want to go this route, you can also use individual silicone baking cups.

Parchment. Specially pre-cut parchment can be helpful to making cleanup even easier when baking with your air fryer. Additionally, you can find parchment paper with precut holes for easy steaming.

Pizza pan. Yes, you can bake a pizza in your air fryer, and this book includes several recipes for different kinds of keto-friendly pizzas. This is a great option for easily getting the perfect shape every time.

Accessory Removal

At some point you will need to get those helpful accessories out of your air fryer without burning yourself. Here are some tools that will allow you to take items out of your air fryer safely and easily.

Tongs. These will be helpful when lifting meat in and out of the air fryer. Tongs are also helpful for removing cooking pans that don't come with handles.

Oven mitts. Sometimes simple is best. Your food will be very hot when you remove it, so it's great to have these around to protect your hands.

Cleaning Your Air Fryer

Before cleaning it, first ensure that your air fryer is completely cool and unplugged. To clean the air fryer pan you'll need to:

1. Remove the air fryer pan from the base. Fill the pan with hot water and dish soap. Let the pan soak with the frying basket inside for 10 minutes.
2. Then clean the basket thoroughly with a sponge or brush.
3. Remove the fryer basket and scrub the underside and outside walls.
4. Clean the air fryer pan with a sponge or brush.
5. Let everything air-dry and return to the air fryer base.

To clean the outside of your air fryer simply wipe the outside with a damp cloth. Then, be sure all components are in the correct position before beginning your next cooking adventure.

What Is Keto?

The ketogenic diet, or keto, is a very low-carb, moderate-protein, and high-fat diet that allows the body to fuel itself without the use of glucose or high levels of carbohydrates. When the body is in short supply of glucose, ketones are made in the liver from the breakdown of fats through a process called *ketosis*. (Please note this differs from ketoacidosis.) With careful tracking, creative meals, and self-control, this diet can lead to weight loss, lower blood sugar, regulated insulin levels, and controlled cravings.

When you eat a very high-carb diet (pizza, pasta, pastries), your body takes those carbs and turns them into glucose to power itself. When you cut out the carbs, your metabolism burns fat instead. Typically, a ketogenic diet restricts carbs to 0–50 grams per day.

What Are Macros?

Macronutrients, or macros, are the three ways your body produces energy. They include carbohydrates, protein, and fat. When you're following keto, it is very important to track how many grams of each macronutrient you consume each day.

- Carbs should be around 5 percent of your daily calories
- Protein should be around 25 percent of your daily calories
- Healthy fats should be around 70 percent of your daily calories

Some of the best-quality fats come from natural sources such as fish, avocados, and nuts. These fats can help reduce your cholesterol, keep your heart strong, and fuel your body throughout the day. You should always beware of unhealthy fats, however, that can come from foods like cookies and French fries. Overconsumption of these, especially in conjunction with a high-carb diet, can contribute to heart disease, low energy, and unwanted weight gain.

Net Carbs

Most people following keto opt to track net carbs instead of total carbs. You can figure out net carbs by subtracting your dietary fiber intake from your total carb intake:

Total carbs minus dietary fiber equals net carbs

You may also subtract sugar alcohols from the total carb count. Net is generally the preferred method because of how your body reacts to the fiber and sugar alcohols. On nutrition labels, the grams of dietary fiber and sugar alcohols are already included in the total carb count, but because fiber and (some) sugar alcohols are carbs that your body can't digest, they have no effect on your blood sugar levels and can be subtracted.

Tips to Remember

Keep these tips in mind as you plan your daily meals:

Carbs are a limit: Don't go above your allotted daily net carbs.

Protein is a goal: This is the most important macro to hit. If you're losing weight, you want to make sure you're eating enough protein to keep you from also losing muscle.

Fat is a lever—(you use it to adjust your diet): In this diet, fat is designed to keep you full. If you're hungry, go ahead and eat that healthy fat up to your limit. If you're not hungry, you don't have to hit your fat macros.

With the quick and easy recipes in this book, you should never feel deprived on your keto journey. Just remember, if you fall off the wagon, the most important thing is to get back on as quickly as possible. Allow yourself grace and time, but never give up just because you slipped up.

Now that you have a better understanding of your air fryer and the ketogenic diet, let's get cooking! You'll find plenty of recipes to suit all tastes. Use these recipes as a guide and always feel free to season intuitively and customize dishes to your liking, but be aware that doing so will change the provided nutritional stats.

2

Breakfast

Quick and delicious low-carb breakfasts will soon be the norm in your household once you put your air fryer to work! These recipes will kick-start your day in a healthy way without depriving you of the savory goodness mornings should be made of! When you're struggling to get out the door in time, it can be really tough to prepare a nourishing meal for yourself or your family. Grabbing a granola bar or toaster pastry may be the easiest option, but it can soon lead to feelings of guilt and serious midday hunger.

The recipes in this chapter are filling and keto-approved, helping you to change your mornings and your entire days. Get ready for nutritious breakfasts that can be made in a flash. With meals you can prepare ahead of time, like Sausage and Cheese Balls, and dishes you can pop in your air fryer to get ready while you get ready, like Quick and Easy Bacon Strips, you'll wish you had started air frying your breakfasts sooner!

Crunchy Granola

Missing the crunch of cereal in the morning? This recipe saves the day in a simple way because making it is as easy as mixing all the ingredients together and popping it in your air fryer! Once the granola is done, you can enjoy it in a bowl of unsweetened nut milk or on top of a low-carb, full-fat yogurt!

- **Hands-On Time: 10 minutes**
- **Cook Time: 5 minutes**

Serves 6

2 cups pecans, chopped

1 cup unsweetened coconut flakes

1 cup almond slivers

⅓ cup sunflower seeds

¼ cup golden flaxseed

¼ cup low-carb, sugar-free chocolate chips

¼ cup granular erythritol

2 tablespoons unsalted butter

1 teaspoon ground cinnamon

WAYS TO ENJOY

You can enjoy this granola with a bowl of unsweetened almond milk, or make it a parfait by mixing up a keto "faux-gurt" made simply of ½ cup sour cream, 1 tablespoon heavy cream, and 1 tablespoon of your favorite low-carb sweetener!

1 In a large bowl, mix all ingredients.

2 Place the mixture into a 4-cup round baking dish. Place dish into the air fryer basket.

3 Adjust the temperature to 320°F and set the timer for 5 minutes.

4 Allow to cool completely before serving.

PER SERVING

CALORIES: 617	**FAT:** 55.8 g
PROTEIN: 10.9 g	**SODIUM:** 5 mg
FIBER: 11.2 g	**CARBOHYDRATES:** 32.4 g
NET CARBOHYDRATES: 6.5 g	**SUGAR:** 2.7 g
SUGAR ALCOHOL: 14.7 g	

Jalapeño Popper Egg Cups

The savory goodness of this classic appetizer has finally come to breakfast! Spice up your morning with eggs that pack a serious punch and crunch! Be sure to make enough for second helpings...you'll be glad you did!

- **Hands-On Time: 10 minutes**
- **Cook Time: 10 minutes**

Serves 2

4 large eggs

¼ cup chopped pickled jalapeños

2 ounces full-fat cream cheese

½ cup shredded sharp Cheddar cheese

1 In a medium bowl, beat the eggs, then pour into four silicone muffin cups.

2 In a large microwave-safe bowl, place jalapeños, cream cheese, and Cheddar. Microwave for 30 seconds and stir. Take a spoonful, approximately ¼ of the mixture, and place it in the center of one of the egg cups. Repeat with remaining mixture.

3 Place egg cups into the air fryer basket.

4 Adjust the temperature to 320°F and set the timer for 10 minutes.

5 Serve warm.

PER SERVING

CALORIES: 354	FAT: 25.3 g
PROTEIN: 21.0 g	SODIUM: 601 mg
FIBER: 0.2 g	CARBOHYDRATES: 2.3 g
NET CARBOHYDRATES: 2.1 g	SUGAR: 1.4 g

Crispy Southwestern Ham Egg Cups

This recipe, cooked right in the cups lined with delicious ham, will start your day with a burst of creamy, subtly spicy Southwestern flavor. The sour cream in the dish helps cut the spice and adds fat to your meal that helps keep you full!

- **Hands-On Time: 5 minutes**
- **Cook Time: 12 minutes**

Serves 2

4 (1-ounce) slices deli ham

4 large eggs

2 tablespoons full-fat sour cream

¼ cup diced green bell pepper

2 tablespoons diced red bell pepper

2 tablespoons diced white onion

½ cup shredded medium Cheddar cheese

1 Place one slice of ham on the bottom of four baking cups.

2 In a large bowl, whisk eggs with sour cream. Stir in green pepper, red pepper, and onion.

3 Pour the egg mixture into ham-lined baking cups. Top with Cheddar. Place cups into the air fryer basket.

4 Adjust the temperature to 320°F and set the timer for 12 minutes or until the tops are browned.

5 Serve warm.

PER SERVING

CALORIES: 382	FAT: 23.6 g
PROTEIN: 29.4 g	SODIUM: 977 mg
FIBER: 1.4 g	CARBOHYDRATES: 6.0 g
NET CARBOHYDRATES: 4.6 g	SUGAR: 2.1 g

Buffalo Egg Cups

Looking for a great way to take your morning eggs to the next level while packing in an extra boost of protein? These Buffalo Egg Cups are your answer. The spicy buffalo sauce will satisfy your palate, and the eggs' fat and protein will work together to keep you full!

- **Hands-On Time: 10 minutes**
- **Cook Time: 15 minutes**

Serves 2

4 large eggs

2 ounces full-fat cream cheese

2 tablespoons buffalo sauce

½ cup shredded sharp Cheddar cheese

1 Crack eggs into two (4") ramekins.

2 In a small microwave-safe bowl, mix cream cheese, buffalo sauce, and Cheddar. Microwave for 20 seconds and then stir. Place a spoonful into each ramekin on top of the eggs.

3 Place ramekins into the air fryer basket.

4 Adjust the temperature to 320°F and set the timer for 15 minutes.

5 Serve warm.

PER SERVING

CALORIES: 354

PROTEIN: 21.0 g

FIBER: 0.0 g

NET CARBOHYDRATES: 2.3 g

FAT: 22.3 g

SODIUM: 886 mg

CARBOHYDRATES: 2.3 g

SUGAR: 1.4 g

Veggie Frittata

Want to get your day started with a nutritious and filling boost? This breakfast is just what you need to help you get your daily veggies in early! Of course vegetables are packed with nutrients to help keep you healthy and strong, but it's important to keep an eye on the carb counts because vegetables have a huge range.

- **Hands-On Time: 15 minutes**
- **Cook Time: 12 minutes**

Serves 4

6 large eggs
¼ cup heavy whipping cream
½ cup chopped broccoli
¼ cup chopped yellow onion
¼ cup chopped green bell pepper

1 In a large bowl, whisk eggs and heavy whipping cream. Mix in broccoli, onion, and bell pepper.

2 Pour into a 6″ round oven-safe baking dish. Place baking dish into the air fryer basket.

3 Adjust the temperature to 350°F and set the timer for 12 minutes.

4 Eggs should be firm and cooked fully when the frittata is done. Serve warm.

PER SERVING

CALORIES: 168	**FAT:** 11.8 g
PROTEIN: 10.2 g	**SODIUM:** 116 mg
FIBER: 0.6 g	**CARBOHYDRATES:** 3.1 g
NET CARBOHYDRATES: 2.5 g	**SUGAR:** 1.5 g

Pumpkin Spice Muffins

Who doesn't love the taste of pumpkin on a crisp autumn morning? For most people, pumpkin and fall go hand in hand, and this recipe will be a staple in your breakfast rotation all season long!

- **Hands-On Time: 10 minutes**
- **Cook Time: 15 minutes**

Serves 6

1 cup blanched finely ground almond flour
½ cup granular erythritol
½ teaspoon baking powder
¼ cup unsalted butter, softened
¼ cup pure pumpkin purée
½ teaspoon ground cinnamon
¼ teaspoon ground nutmeg
1 teaspoon vanilla extract
2 large eggs

READ YOUR LABELS!

Make sure you use regular pumpkin purée instead of pumpkin pie purée! It can be tricky because they're usually right next to each other on store shelves, but the latter has added carbs and sugar that you definitely don't need for this flavorful treat!

1 In a large bowl, mix almond flour, erythritol, baking powder, butter, pumpkin purée, cinnamon, nutmeg, and vanilla.

2 Gently stir in eggs.

3 Evenly pour the batter into six silicone muffin cups. Place muffin cups into the air fryer basket, working in batches if necessary.

4 Adjust the temperature to 300°F and set the timer for 15 minutes.

5 When completely cooked, a toothpick inserted in center will come out mostly clean. Serve warm.

PER SERVING

CALORIES: 205
PROTEIN: 6.3 g
FIBER: 2.4 g
NET CARBOHYDRATES: 3.0 g
SUGAR ALCOHOL: 12.0 g

FAT: 18.0 g
SODIUM: 65 mg
CARBOHYDRATES: 17.4 g
SUGAR: 1.3 g

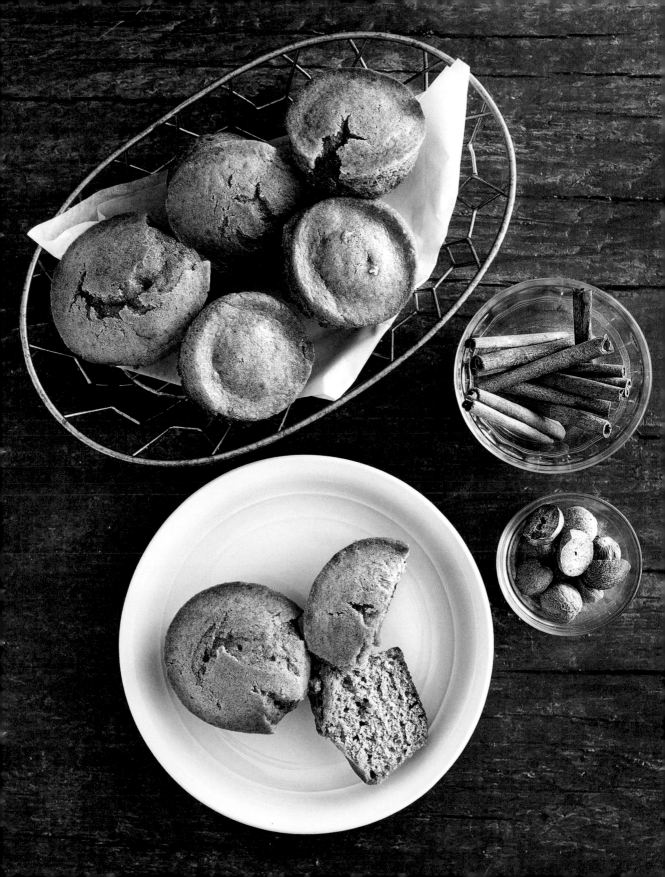

Quick and Easy Bacon Strips

What's better than perfectly crisped bacon in the morning? Gone are the days of cautiously standing over a hot pan while grease splatters at you. With your air fryer, you're just minutes away from delicious strips of evenly cooked bacon every time!

- **Hands-On Time: 5 minutes**
- **Cook Time: 12 minutes**

Serves 4

8 slices sugar-free bacon

1 Place bacon strips into the air fryer basket.

2 Adjust the temperature to 400°F and set the timer for 12 minutes.

3 After 6 minutes, flip bacon and continue cooking time. Serve warm.

PER SERVING

CALORIES: 88	**FAT:** 6.2 g
PROTEIN: 5.8 g	**SODIUM:** 355 mg
FIBER: 0.0 g	**CARBOHYDRATES:** 0.2 g
NET CARBOHYDRATES: 0.2 g	**SUGAR:** 0.0 g

"Banana" Nut Cake

Even though bananas aren't a great option for keto because of high carb count, you can still enjoy banana nut cake by employing the help of the very low-carb banana extract. You can customize these muffins to your liking by swapping out the walnuts for your favorite nut.

- **Hands-On Time: 15 minutes**
- **Cook Time: 25 minutes**

Serves 6

1 cup blanched finely ground almond flour
½ cup powdered erythritol
2 tablespoons ground golden flaxseed
2 teaspoons baking powder
½ teaspoon ground cinnamon
¼ cup unsalted butter, melted
2½ teaspoons banana extract
1 teaspoon vanilla extract
¼ cup full-fat sour cream
2 large eggs
¼ cup chopped walnuts

WHY NOT REAL BANANAS?

One medium banana has about 24 grams of net carbohydrates. That's more than you would probably eat in a whole day! Banana extract is an excellent replacement that can be found in your local grocery store.

1. In a large bowl, mix almond flour, erythritol, flaxseed, baking powder, and cinnamon.

2. Stir in butter, banana extract, vanilla extract, and sour cream.

3. Add eggs to the mixture and gently stir until fully combined. Stir in the walnuts.

4. Pour into 6" nonstick cake pan and place into the air fryer basket.

5. Adjust the temperature to 300°F and set the timer for 25 minutes.

6. Cake will be golden and a toothpick inserted in center will come out clean when fully cooked. Allow to fully cool to avoid crumbling.

PER SERVING

CALORIES: 263	**FAT:** 23.6 g
PROTEIN: 7.6 g	**SODIUM:** 192 mg
FIBER: 3.1 g	**CARBOHYDRATES:** 18.4 g
NET CARBOHYDRATES: 3.3 g	**SUGAR:** 1.3 g
SUGAR ALCOHOL: 12.0 g	

Lemon Poppy Seed Cake

You can set this cake cooking when you get up in the morning, hop in the shower, and return to a moist and delicious low-carb treat that will be hard to put down! It's a great way to get your day started with a smile on your face!

- **Hands-On Time: 10 minutes**
- **Cook Time: 14 minutes**

Serves 6

1 cup blanched finely ground almond flour

½ cup powdered erythritol

½ teaspoon baking powder

¼ cup unsalted butter, melted

¼ cup unsweetened almond milk

2 large eggs

1 teaspoon vanilla extract

1 medium lemon

1 teaspoon poppy seeds

1 In a large bowl, mix almond flour, erythritol, baking powder, butter, almond milk, eggs, and vanilla.

2 Slice the lemon in half and squeeze the juice into a small bowl, then add to the batter.

3 Using a fine grater, zest the lemon and add 1 tablespoon zest to the batter and stir. Add poppy seeds to batter.

4 Pour batter into nonstick 6" round cake pan. Place pan into the air fryer basket.

5 Adjust the temperature to 300°F and set the timer for 14 minutes.

6 When fully cooked, a toothpick inserted in center will come out mostly clean. The cake will finish cooking and firm up as it cools. Serve at room temperature.

PER SERVING

CALORIES: 204	**FAT:** 18.2 g
PROTEIN: 6.3 g	**SODIUM:** 72 mg
FIBER: 2.4 g	**CARBOHYDRATES:** 16.9 g
NET CARBOHYDRATES: 2.5 g	**SUGAR:** 0.9 g
SUGAR ALCOHOL: 12.0 g	

Pancake Cake

This bakes up quick for a fluffy and delicious breakfast for the whole family. It's a treat that the kids will love, and you'll love how simple it is to make! For added fun, you can throw in a handful of low-carb chocolate chips! Serve this with low-carb syrup or sugar-free whipped cream and low-carb berries such as strawberries or blackberries.

- **Hands-On Time: 10 minutes**
- **Cook Time: 7 minutes**

Serves 4

½ cup blanched finely ground almond flour

¼ cup powdered erythritol

½ teaspoon baking powder

2 tablespoons unsalted butter, softened

1 large egg

½ teaspoon unflavored gelatin

½ teaspoon vanilla extract

½ teaspoon ground cinnamon

1 In a large bowl, mix almond flour, erythritol, and baking powder. Add butter, egg, gelatin, vanilla, and cinnamon. Pour into 6" round baking pan.

2 Place pan into the air fryer basket.

3 Adjust the temperature to 300°F and set the timer for 7 minutes.

4 When the cake is completely cooked, a toothpick will come out clean. Cut cake into four and serve.

PER SERVING

CALORIES: 153	**FAT:** 13.4 g
PROTEIN: 5.4 g	**SODIUM:** 80 mg
FIBER: 1.7 g	**CARBOHYDRATES:** 12.6 g
NET CARBOHYDRATES: 1.9 g	**SUGAR:** 0.6 g
SUGAR ALCOHOL: 9.0 g	

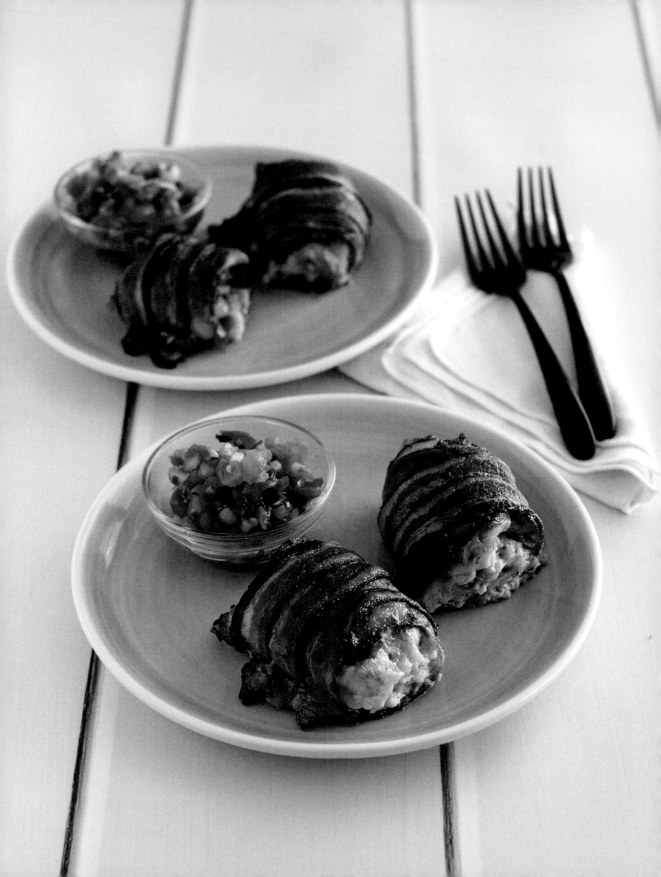

Bacon, Egg, and Cheese Roll Ups

This is the tastiest spin on a breakfast burrito you've ever tried! With all of the carbs in a regular tortilla, why not just replace the wrap altogether with crispy and savory bacon? Load your burrito up with all the goods, and pick it up just like the classic version!

- **Hands-On Time: 15 minutes**
- **Cook Time: 15 minutes**

Serves 4

2 tablespoons unsalted butter

¼ cup chopped onion

½ medium green bell pepper, seeded and chopped

6 large eggs

12 slices sugar-free bacon

1 cup shredded sharp Cheddar cheese

½ cup mild salsa, for dipping

MAKE IT YOUR OWN!

Customize this dish with your favorite egg add-ins! Chopped onions, mushrooms, or spinach are all great low-carb options. If you're extra hungry, adding some cooked crumbled breakfast sausage will make this even more filling!

1 In a medium skillet over medium heat, melt butter. Add onion and pepper to the skillet and sauté until fragrant and onions are translucent, about 3 minutes.

2 Whisk eggs in a small bowl and pour into skillet. Scramble eggs with onions and peppers until fluffy and fully cooked, about 5 minutes. Remove from heat and set aside.

3 On work surface, place three slices of bacon side by side, overlapping about ¼". Place ¼ cup scrambled eggs in a heap on the side closest to you and sprinkle ¼ cup cheese on top of the eggs.

4 Tightly roll the bacon around the eggs and secure the seam with a toothpick if necessary. Place each roll into the air fryer basket.

5 Adjust the temperature to 350°F and set the timer for 15 minutes. Rotate the rolls halfway through the cooking time.

6 Bacon will be brown and crispy when completely cooked. Serve immediately with salsa for dipping.

PER SERVING

CALORIES: 460	**FAT:** 31.7 g
PROTEIN: 28.2 g	**SODIUM:** 1,100 mg
FIBER: 0.8 g	**CARBOHYDRATES:** 6.1 g
NET CARBOHYDRATES: 5.3 g	**SUGAR:** 3.1 g

Cheesy Cauliflower Hash Browns

Because high-carb potatoes aren't a good option for keto, cauliflower makes a great nutrient-dense, low-carb substitute for hash browns. And with the help of your air fryer, you can get them perfectly crispy in no time at all! The cheese in this recipe helps bind the cauliflower together and adds an irresistible flavor that your whole family will love!

- **Hands-On Time: 20 minutes**
- **Cook Time: 12 minutes**

Serves 4

1 (12-ounce) steamer bag cauliflower
1 large egg
1 cup shredded sharp Cheddar cheese

1 Place bag in microwave and cook according to package instructions. Allow to cool completely and put cauliflower into a cheesecloth or kitchen towel and squeeze to remove excess moisture.

2 Mash cauliflower with a fork and add egg and cheese.

3 Cut a piece of parchment to fit your air fryer basket. Take ¼ of the mixture and form it into a hash brown patty shape. Place it onto the parchment and into the air fryer basket, working in batches if necessary.

4 Adjust the temperature to 400°F and set the timer for 12 minutes.

5 Flip the hash browns halfway through the cooking time. When completely cooked, they will be golden brown. Serve immediately.

PER SERVING

CALORIES: 153	**FAT:** 9.5 g
PROTEIN: 10.0 g	**SODIUM:** 225 mg
FIBER: 1.7 g	**CARBOHYDRATES:** 4.7 g
NET CARBOHYDRATES: 3.0 g	**SUGAR:** 1.8 g

Breakfast Stuffed Poblanos

Get ready for a brand-new breakfast in your weekly rotation. This morning spin on jalapeño poppers will give you the kick you need to start your day. Crisped perfectly in your air fryer, this will also become a favorite for those "breakfast for dinner" nights!

- **Hands-On Time: 15 minutes**
- **Cook Time: 15 minutes**

Serves 4

½ pound spicy ground pork breakfast sausage

4 large eggs

4 ounces full-fat cream cheese, softened

¼ cup canned diced tomatoes and green chiles, drained

4 large poblano peppers

8 tablespoons shredded pepper jack cheese

½ cup full-fat sour cream

1 In a medium skillet over medium heat, crumble and brown the ground sausage until no pink remains. Remove sausage and drain the fat from the pan. Crack eggs into the pan, scramble, and cook until no longer runny.

2 Place cooked sausage in a large bowl and fold in cream cheese. Mix in diced tomatoes and chiles. Gently fold in eggs.

3 Cut a 4"–5" slit in the top of each poblano, removing the seeds and white membrane with a small knife. Separate the filling into four servings and spoon carefully into each pepper. Top each with 2 tablespoons pepper jack cheese.

4 Place each pepper into the air fryer basket.

5 Adjust the temperature to 350°F and set the timer for 15 minutes.

6 Peppers will be soft and cheese will be browned when ready. Serve immediately with sour cream on top.

PER SERVING

CALORIES: 489

PROTEIN: 22.8 g

FIBER: 3.8 g

NET CARBOHYDRATES: 8.8 g

FAT: 35.6 g

SODIUM: 746 mg

CARBOHYDRATES: 12.6 g

SUGAR: 2.9 g

Air Fryer "Hard-Boiled" Eggs

Yes, it is possible to "hard-boil" whole eggs in your air fryer! This method may seem a bit out of the ordinary, but it's a great way to achieve the same results you're used to without having to boil a pot of water on the stove! This is the perfect way to prepare several grab-and-go snacks to support your ketogenic lifestyle.

- **Hands-On Time: 2 minutes**
- **Cook Time: 18 minutes**

Serves 4

4 large eggs
1 cup water

AIR-BOILED EGGS?

Of course there are other ways to get perfect hard-boiled eggs, but your air fryer is a great low-energy option. If you don't have room on your stove, this is the perfect way to cook several eggs at once.

1 Place eggs into a 4-cup round baking-safe dish and pour water over eggs. Place dish into the air fryer basket.

2 Adjust the temperature to 300°F and set the timer for 18 minutes.

3 Store cooked eggs in the refrigerator until ready to use or peel and eat warm.

PER SERVING

CALORIES: 77	FAT: 4.4 g
PROTEIN: 6.3 g	SODIUM: 62 mg
FIBER: 0.0 g	CARBOHYDRATES: 0.6 g
NET CARBOHYDRATES: 0.6 g	SUGAR: 0.6 g

Scrambled Eggs

Sometimes you just don't want to turn on your stove, or you don't have access to it for whatever reason. When you're in a pinch, you can still get classic moist Scrambled Eggs from your air fryer!

- **Hands-On Time: 5 minutes**
- **Cook Time: 15 minutes**

Serves 2

4 large eggs
2 tablespoons unsalted
   butter, melted
½ cup shredded sharp
   Cheddar cheese

1 Crack eggs into 2-cup round baking dish and whisk. Place dish into the air fryer basket.

2 Adjust the temperature to 400°F and set the timer for 10 minutes.

3 After 5 minutes, stir the eggs and add the butter and cheese. Let cook 3 more minutes and stir again.

4 Allow eggs to finish cooking an additional 2 minutes or remove if they are to your desired liking.

5 Use a fork to fluff. Serve warm.

PER SERVING

CALORIES: 359
PROTEIN: 19.5 g
FIBER: 0.0 g
NET CARBOHYDRATES: 1.1 g

FAT: 27.6 g
SODIUM: 325 mg
CARBOHYDRATES: 1.1 g
SUGAR: 0.5 g

Loaded Cauliflower Breakfast Bake

Casseroles aren't just for dinnertime! This is the perfect option for busy weekday mornings, giving you lots of classic breakfast flavor and swapping in cauliflower where potatoes might usually be. Add a dash of hot sauce for some kick if you really want to wake up!

- **Hands-On Time: 15 minutes**
- **Cook Time: 20 minutes**

Serves 4

6 large eggs

¼ cup heavy whipping cream

1½ cups chopped cauliflower

1 cup shredded medium Cheddar cheese

1 medium avocado, peeled and pitted

8 tablespoons full-fat sour cream

2 scallions, sliced on the bias

12 slices sugar-free bacon, cooked and crumbled

1 In a medium bowl, whisk eggs and cream together. Pour into a 4-cup round baking dish.

2 Add cauliflower and mix, then top with Cheddar. Place dish into the air fryer basket.

3 Adjust the temperature to 320°F and set the timer for 20 minutes.

4 When completely cooked, eggs will be firm and cheese will be browned. Slice into four pieces.

5 Slice avocado and divide evenly among pieces. Top each piece with 2 tablespoons sour cream, sliced scallions, and crumbled bacon.

PER SERVING

CALORIES: 512	**FAT:** 38.3 g
PROTEIN: 27.1 g	**SODIUM:** 865 mg
FIBER: 3.2 g	**CARBOHYDRATES:** 7.5 g
NET CARBOHYDRATES: 4.3 g	**SUGAR:** 2.3 g

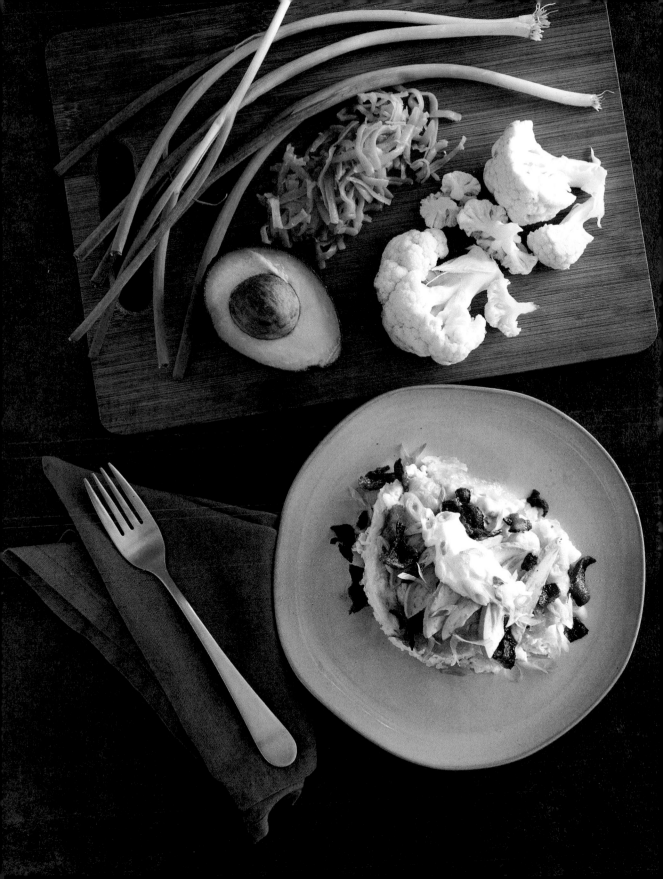

Cinnamon Roll Sticks

With sweet and gooey cinnamon perfection, you'll have a rich start to your morning and guaranteed trouble sharing these Cinnamon Roll Sticks!

- **Hands-On Time: 10 minutes**
- **Cook Time: 7 minutes**

Serves 4 (2 sticks per serving)

1 cup shredded mozzarella cheese

1 ounce full-fat cream cheese

⅓ cup blanched finely ground almond flour

½ teaspoon baking soda

½ cup granular erythritol, divided

1 teaspoon vanilla extract

1 large egg

2 tablespoons unsalted butter, melted

½ teaspoon ground cinnamon

3 tablespoons powdered erythritol

2 teaspoons unsweetened vanilla almond milk

1 Place mozzarella in a large microwave-safe bowl and break cream cheese into small pieces and place into bowl. Microwave for 45 seconds.

2 Stir in almond flour, baking soda, ¼ cup granular erythritol, and vanilla. A soft dough should form. Microwave the mix for additional 15 seconds if it becomes too stiff.

3 Mix egg into the dough, using your hands if necessary.

4 Cut a piece of parchment to fit your air fryer basket. Press the dough into an 8″ × 5″ rectangle on the parchment and cut into eight (1″) sticks.

5 In a small bowl, mix butter, cinnamon, and remaining granular erythritol. Brush half the mixture over the top of the sticks and place them into the air fryer basket.

6 Adjust the temperature to 400°F and set the timer for 7 minutes.

7 Halfway through the cooking time, flip the sticks and brush with remaining butter mixture. When done, sticks should be crispy.

8 To make glaze, whisk powdered erythritol and almond milk in a small bowl. Drizzle over cinnamon sticks. Serve warm.

PER SERVING

CALORIES: 233	**FAT:** 19.0 g
PROTEIN: 10.3 g	**SODIUM:** 378 mg
FIBER: 1.2 g	**CARBOHYDRATES:** 40.2 g
NET CARBOHYDRATES: 2.2 g	**SUGAR:** 1.0 g
SUGAR ALCOHOL: 36.8 g	

Breakfast Calzone

This is a great, and portable, way to start your morning! You can customize the filling with all of your favorites, freeze it the night before, and warm it up in your air fryer before taking it with you on your morning commute!

- **Hands-On Time: 15 minutes**
- **Cook Time: 15 minutes**

Serves 4

1½ cups shredded mozzarella cheese

½ cup blanched finely ground almond flour

1 ounce full-fat cream cheese

1 large whole egg

4 large eggs, scrambled

½ pound cooked breakfast sausage, crumbled

8 tablespoons shredded mild Cheddar cheese

1. In a large microwave-safe bowl, add mozzarella, almond flour, and cream cheese. Microwave for 1 minute. Stir until the mixture is smooth and forms a ball. Add the egg and stir until dough forms.

2. Place dough between two sheets of parchment and roll out to ¼" thickness. Cut the dough into four rectangles.

3. Mix scrambled eggs and cooked sausage together in a large bowl. Divide the mixture evenly among each piece of dough, placing it on the lower half of the rectangle. Sprinkle each with 2 tablespoons Cheddar.

4. Fold over the rectangle to cover the egg and meat mixture. Pinch, roll, or use a wet fork to close the edges completely.

5. Cut a piece of parchment to fit your air fryer basket and place the calzones onto the parchment. Place parchment into the air fryer basket.

6. Adjust the temperature to 380°F and set the timer for 15 minutes.

7. Flip the calzones halfway through the cooking time. When done, calzones should be golden in color. Serve immediately.

PER SERVING

CALORIES: 560	**FAT:** 41.7 g
PROTEIN: 34.5 g	**SODIUM:** 930 mg
FIBER: 1.5 g	**CARBOHYDRATES:** 5.7 g
NET CARBOHYDRATES: 4.2 g	**SUGAR:** 2.1 g

Cauliflower Avocado Toast

Disappointed you can't keep up with the trend of avocado toast? Have no fear, this swap is a tasty, crunchy nutrient-rich breakfast that's full of healthy fats to help keep you full and focused throughout the day!

- **Hands-On Time: 15 minutes**
- **Cook Time: 8 minutes**

Serves 2

1 (12-ounce) steamer bag cauliflower
1 large egg
½ cup shredded mozzarella cheese
1 ripe medium avocado
½ teaspoon garlic powder
¼ teaspoon ground black pepper

1 Cook cauliflower according to package instructions. Remove from bag and place into cheesecloth or clean towel to remove excess moisture.

2 Place cauliflower into a large bowl and mix in egg and mozzarella. Cut a piece of parchment to fit your air fryer basket. Separate the cauliflower mixture into two, and place it on the parchment in two mounds. Press out the cauliflower mounds into a ¼"-thick rectangle. Place the parchment into the air fryer basket.

3 Adjust the temperature to 400°F and set the timer for 8 minutes.

4 Flip the cauliflower halfway through the cooking time.

5 When the timer beeps, remove the parchment and allow the cauliflower to cool 5 minutes.

6 Cut open the avocado and remove the pit. Scoop out the inside, place it in a medium bowl, and mash it with garlic powder and pepper. Spread onto the cauliflower. Serve immediately.

PER SERVING

CALORIES: 278	**FAT:** 15.6 g
PROTEIN: 14.1 g	**SODIUM:** 267 mg
FIBER: 8.2 g	**CARBOHYDRATES:** 15.9 g
NET CARBOHYDRATES: 7.7 g	**SUGAR:** 3.9 g

Sausage and Cheese Balls

These breakfast-style meatballs make for a flavorful, protein-filled breakfast that you can make ahead of time, freeze, and pop into your air fryer when you're ready so your busy mornings are easy and delicious!

- **Hands-On Time: 10 minutes**
- **Cook Time: 12 minutes**

Yields 16 balls (4 per serving)

1 pound pork breakfast
    sausage
½ cup shredded Cheddar
    cheese
1 ounce full-fat cream
    cheese, softened
1 large egg

FREEZER FRIENDLY!
These cheese balls are a great make-ahead item. If you want to freeze them, place cooked balls on a large cookie sheet and freeze for 1 hour. Then place in a freezer-safe storage bag.

1 Mix all ingredients in a large bowl. Form into sixteen (1″) balls. Place the balls into the air fryer basket.

2 Adjust the temperature to 400°F and set the timer for 12 minutes.

3 Shake the basket two or three times during cooking. Sausage balls will be browned on the outside and have an internal temperature of at least 145°F when completely cooked.

4 Serve warm.

PER SERVING

CALORIES: 424	**FAT:** 32.2 g
PROTEIN: 22.8 g	**SODIUM:** 973 mg
FIBER: 0.0 g	**CARBOHYDRATES:** 1.6 g
NET CARBOHYDRATES: 1.6 g	**SUGAR:** 1.4 g

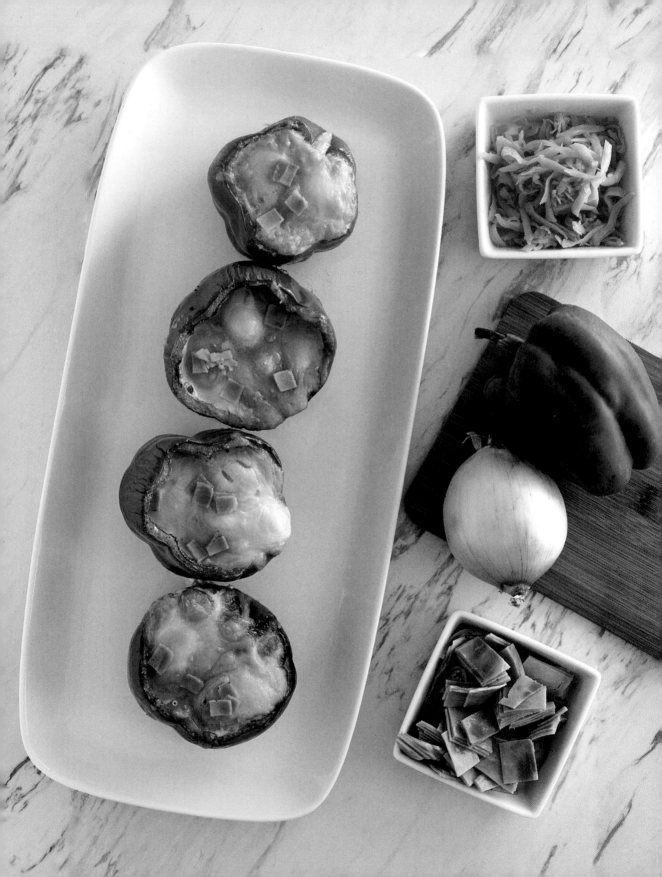

Cheesy Bell Pepper Eggs

Bell peppers are a great source of vitamins A and C, two vitamins that are important for the strength of your immune system. This easy breakfast also gives you some protein from the ham and an extra boost of flavor from the onion. Altogether, you have a nutritious, well-rounded breakfast!

- **Hands-On Time: 10 minutes**
- **Cook Time: 15 minutes**

Serves 4

4 medium green bell peppers

3 ounces cooked ham, chopped

¼ medium onion, peeled and chopped

8 large eggs

1 cup mild Cheddar cheese

1 Cut the tops off each bell pepper. Remove the seeds and the white membranes with a small knife. Place ham and onion into each pepper.

2 Crack 2 eggs into each pepper. Top with ¼ cup cheese per pepper. Place into the air fryer basket.

3 Adjust the temperature to 390°F and set the timer for 15 minutes.

4 When fully cooked, peppers will be tender and eggs will be firm. Serve immediately.

PER SERVING

CALORIES: 314	FAT: 18.6 g
PROTEIN: 24.9 g	SODIUM: 621 mg
FIBER: 1.7 g	CARBOHYDRATES: 6.3 g
NET CARBOHYDRATES: 4.6 g	SUGAR: 3.0 g

Spaghetti Squash Fritters

Squash is very quick to cook in the air fryer and has so many uses beyond just savory dinners. This dish is surprisingly flavorful and a breeze to make. Feel free to customize to your liking by adding your favorite filling items, such as mushrooms, chopped broccoli, or crumbled sausage.

- **Hands-On Time: 15 minutes**
- **Cook Time: 8 minutes**

Serves 4

2 cups cooked spaghetti squash

2 tablespoons unsalted butter, softened

1 large egg

¼ cup blanched finely ground almond flour

2 stalks green onion, sliced

½ teaspoon garlic powder

1 teaspoon dried parsley

1 Remove excess moisture from the squash using a cheesecloth or kitchen towel.

2 Mix all ingredients in a large bowl. Form into four patties.

3 Cut a piece of parchment to fit your air fryer basket. Place each patty on the parchment and place into the air fryer basket.

4 Adjust the temperature to 400°F and set the timer for 8 minutes.

5 Flip the patties halfway through the cooking time. Serve warm.

PER SERVING

CALORIES: 131	**FAT:** 10.1 g
PROTEIN: 3.8 g	**SODIUM:** 33 mg
FIBER: 2.0 g	**CARBOHYDRATES:** 7.1 g
NET CARBOHYDRATES: 5.1 g	**SUGAR:** 2.3 g

3

Appetizers and Snacks

Sometimes appetizers can be more exciting than meals, and all of us have eaten a tray of delicious small bites in place of a meal at least a time or two! That fun cocktail party tradition doesn't have to end just because you're sticking to a low-carb lifestyle. Whether you're hosting an event or just looking for a keto version of your restaurant favorites, the recipes in this chapter like Bacon-Wrapped Jalapeño Poppers and Garlic Cheese Bread will keep you and your guests satisfied without sabotaging your diet!

Prosciutto-Wrapped Parmesan Asparagus

Prosciutto is a thinly sliced Italian ham reminiscent of a less salty bacon. In this recipe it is used to offset the bitterness of asparagus for a more complete and satisfying vegetable appetizer.

- **Hands-On Time: 10 minutes**
- **Cook Time: 10 minutes**

Serves 4

1 pound asparagus

12 (0.5-ounce) slices prosciutto

1 tablespoon coconut oil, melted

2 teaspoons lemon juice

⅛ teaspoon red pepper flakes

⅓ cup grated Parmesan cheese

2 tablespoons salted butter, melted

1 On a clean work surface, place an asparagus spear onto a slice of prosciutto.

2 Drizzle with coconut oil and lemon juice. Sprinkle red pepper flakes and Parmesan across asparagus. Roll prosciutto around asparagus spear. Place into the air fryer basket.

3 Adjust the temperature to 375°F and set the timer for 10 minutes.

4 Drizzle the asparagus roll with butter before serving.

PER SERVING

CALORIES: 263	**FAT:** 20.2 g
PROTEIN: 13.9 g	**SODIUM:** 368 mg
FIBER: 2.4 g	**CARBOHYDRATES:** 6.7 g
NET CARBOHYDRATES: 4.3 g	**SUGAR:** 2.2 g

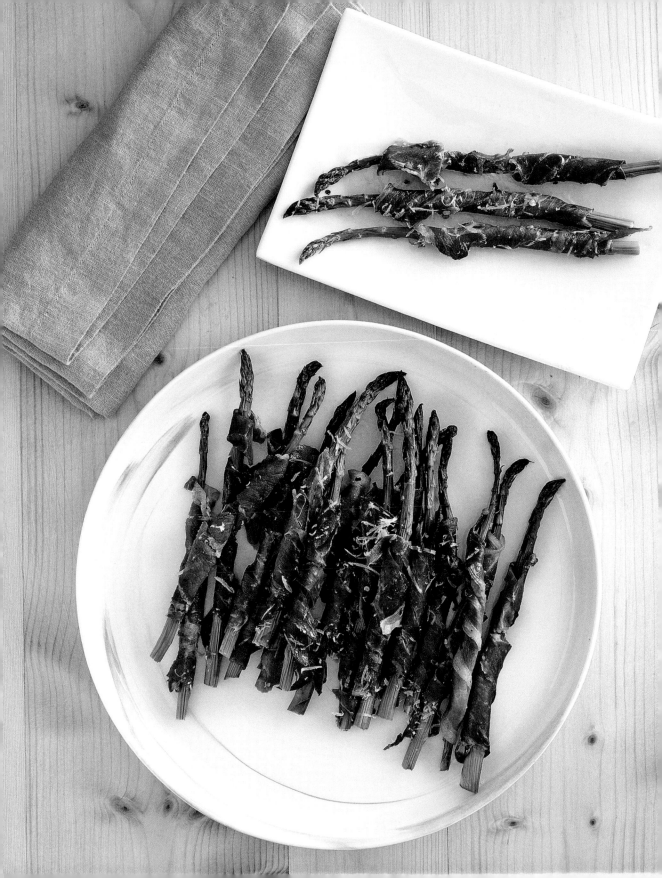

Bacon-Wrapped Jalapeño Poppers

Traditional jalapeño poppers are covered in breading. You won't miss any of that with this spicy and creamy low-carb twist! These irresistible poppers will be a huge hit at your next gathering, and all you'll have to worry about is making sure you brought enough for everyone!

- **Hands-On Time: 15 minutes**
- **Cook Time: 12 minutes**

Serves 4

6 jalapeños (about 4" long each)

3 ounces full-fat cream cheese

⅓ cup shredded medium Cheddar cheese

¼ teaspoon garlic powder

12 slices sugar-free bacon

BE SURE TO WEAR GLOVES!
Use caution when cutting into fresh jalapeños because they contain oils that may act as a skin irritant and cause burning. Using kitchen gloves is a great option to keep the oil off your hands. If you do come into contact with the oil, lemon juice will neutralize the burning.

1 Cut the tops off of the jalapeños and slice down the center lengthwise into two pieces. Use a knife to carefully remove white membrane and seeds from peppers.

2 In a large microwave-safe bowl, place cream cheese, Cheddar, and garlic powder. Microwave for 30 seconds and stir. Spoon cheese mixture into hollow jalapeños.

3 Wrap a slice of bacon around each jalapeño half, completely covering pepper. Place into the air fryer basket.

4 Adjust the temperature to 400°F and set the timer for 12 minutes.

5 Turn the peppers halfway through the cooking time. Serve warm.

PER SERVING

CALORIES: 246	**FAT:** 17.9 g
PROTEIN: 14.4 g	**SODIUM:** 625 mg
FIBER: 0.6 g	**CARBOHYDRATES:** 2.6 g
NET CARBOHYDRATES: 2.0 g	**SUGAR:** 1.6 g

Garlic Parmesan Chicken Wings

Garlic Parmesan is a buttery, cheesy mixture that's a perfect sauce for savory wings. Whether they're for game day with your friends or a company potluck, these wings will be the star of any appetizer tray!

- **Hands-On Time: 5 minutes**
- **Cook Time: 25 minutes**

Serves 4

2 pounds raw chicken wings

1 teaspoon pink Himalayan salt

½ teaspoon garlic powder

1 tablespoon baking powder

4 tablespoons unsalted butter, melted

⅓ cup grated Parmesan cheese

¼ teaspoon dried parsley

1 In a large bowl, place chicken wings, salt, ½ teaspoon garlic powder, and baking powder, then toss. Place wings into the air fryer basket.

2 Adjust the temperature to 400°F and set the timer for 25 minutes.

3 Toss the basket two or three times during the cooking time.

4 In a small bowl, combine butter, Parmesan, and parsley.

5 Remove wings from the fryer and place into a clean large bowl. Pour the butter mixture over the wings and toss until coated. Serve warm.

PER SERVING

CALORIES: 565	**FAT:** 42.1 g
PROTEIN: 41.8 g	**SODIUM:** 1,067 mg
FIBER: 0.1 g	**CARBOHYDRATES:** 2.2 g
NET CARBOHYDRATES: 2.1 g	**SUGAR:** 0.0 g

Spicy Buffalo Chicken Dip

This game day classic packs plenty of protein and serious heat. With just a few simple ingredients, you'll have a gooey, mouthwatering dip to serve as the perfect companion for rooting on your favorite team. Skip the chips and instead dip celery sticks for a glorious and nutritious crunch in every bite!

- **Hands-On Time: 10 minutes**
- **Cook Time: 10 minutes**

Serves 4

1 cup cooked, diced chicken breast

8 ounces full-fat cream cheese, softened

½ cup buffalo sauce

⅓ cup full-fat ranch dressing

⅓ cup chopped pickled jalapeños

1½ cups shredded medium Cheddar cheese, divided

2 scallions, sliced on the bias

1 Place chicken into a large bowl. Add cream cheese, buffalo sauce, and ranch dressing. Stir until the sauces are well mixed and mostly smooth. Fold in jalapeños and 1 cup Cheddar.

2 Pour the mixture into a 4-cup round baking dish and place remaining Cheddar on top. Place dish into the air fryer basket.

3 Adjust the temperature to 350°F and set the timer for 10 minutes.

4 When done, the top will be brown and the dip bubbling. Top with sliced scallions. Serve warm.

PER SERVING

CALORIES: 472

PROTEIN: 25.6 g

FIBER: 0.6 g

NET CARBOHYDRATES: 8.5 g

FAT: 32.0 g

SODIUM: 1,532 mg

CARBOHYDRATES: 9.1 g

SUGAR: 7.4 g

Bacon Jalapeño Cheese Bread

In need of a late-night indulgence that feels like you're cheating on your diet? Your air fryer can help with that! This cheese bread is a savory masterpiece that you won't want to share!

- **Hands-On Time: 10 minutes**
- **Cook Time: 15 minutes**

Yields 8 sticks (2 sticks per serving)

2 cups shredded mozzarella cheese

¼ cup grated Parmesan cheese

¼ cup chopped pickled jalapeños

2 large eggs

4 slices sugar-free bacon, cooked and chopped

1 Mix all ingredients in a large bowl. Cut a piece of parchment to fit your air fryer basket.

2 Dampen your hands with a bit of water and press out the mixture into a circle. You may need to separate this into two smaller cheese breads, depending on the size of your fryer.

3 Place the parchment and cheese bread into the air fryer basket.

4 Adjust the temperature to 320°F and set the timer for 15 minutes.

5 Carefully flip the bread when 5 minutes remain.

6 When fully cooked, the top will be golden brown. Serve warm.

PER SERVING

CALORIES: 273	**FAT:** 18.1 g
PROTEIN: 20.1 g	**SODIUM:** 749 mg
FIBER: 0.1 g	**CARBOHYDRATES:** 2.3 g
NET CARBOHYDRATES: 2.1 g	**SUGAR:** 0.7 g

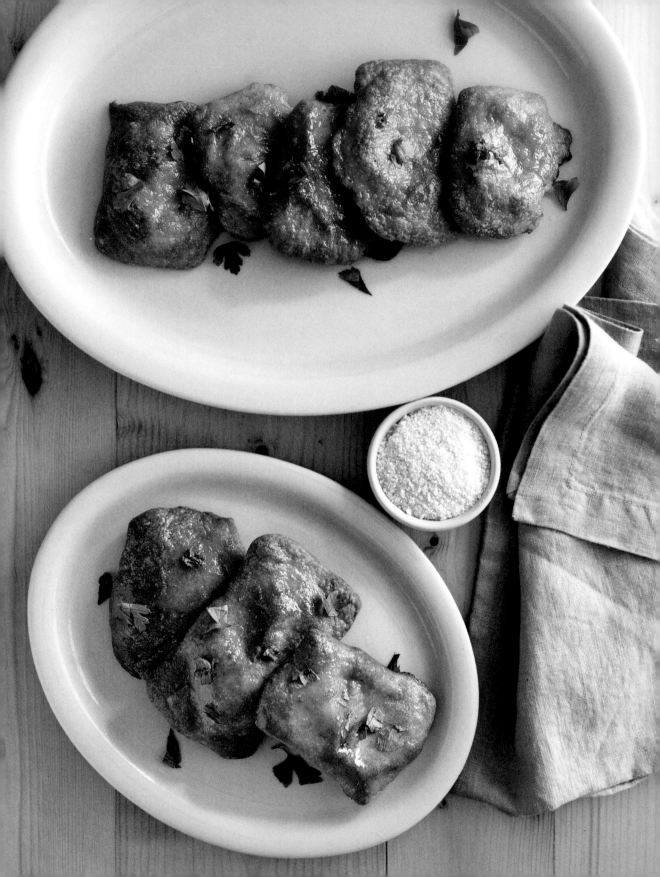

Pizza Rolls

Customize these savory treats with your favorite toppings.

- **Hands-On Time: 15 minutes**
- **Cook Time: 10 minutes**

Yields 24 rolls (3 per serving)

2 cups shredded mozzarella cheese

½ cup almond flour

2 large eggs

72 slices pepperoni

8 (1-ounce) mozzarella string cheese sticks, cut into 3 pieces each

2 tablespoons unsalted butter, melted

¼ teaspoon garlic powder

½ teaspoon dried parsley

2 tablespoons grated Parmesan cheese

1 In a large microwave-safe bowl, place mozzarella and almond flour. Microwave for 1 minute. Remove bowl and mix until ball of dough forms. Microwave additional 30 seconds if necessary.

2 Crack eggs into the bowl and mix until smooth dough ball forms. Wet your hands with water and knead the dough briefly.

3 Tear off two large pieces of parchment paper and spray one side of each with non-stick cooking spray. Place the dough ball between the two sheets, with sprayed sides facing dough. Use a rolling pin to roll dough out to ¼" thickness.

4 Use a knife to slice into 24 rectangles. On each rectangle place 3 pepperoni slices and 1 piece string cheese.

5 Fold the rectangle in half, covering pepperoni and cheese filling. Pinch or roll sides closed. Cut a piece of parchment to fit your air fryer basket and place it into the basket. Put the rolls onto the parchment.

6 Adjust the temperature to 350°F and set the timer for 10 minutes.

7 After 5 minutes, open the fryer and flip the pizza rolls. Restart the fryer and continue cooking until pizza rolls are golden.

8 In a small bowl, place butter, garlic powder, and parsley. Brush the mixture over cooked pizza rolls and then sprinkle with Parmesan. Serve warm.

PER SERVING

CALORIES: 333	**FAT:** 24.0 g
PROTEIN: 20.7 g	**SODIUM:** 708 mg
FIBER: 0.8 g	**CARBOHYDRATES:** 3.3 g
NET CARBOHYDRATES: 2.5 g	**SUGAR:** 0.9 g

Bacon Cheeseburger Dip

This extremely kid-friendly dip is like a burger you can scoop up! It's an ooey-gooey crowd pleaser full of cheesy and savory flavor. Skip the chips and enjoy with pork rinds, or spoon it out onto a fresh romaine lettuce wrap!

- **Hands-On Time: 20 minutes**
- **Cook Time: 10 minutes**

Serves 6

8 ounces full-fat cream cheese

¼ cup full-fat mayonnaise

¼ cup full-fat sour cream

¼ cup chopped onion

1 teaspoon garlic powder

1 tablespoon Worcestershire sauce

1¼ cups shredded medium Cheddar cheese, divided

½ pound cooked 80/20 ground beef

6 slices sugar-free bacon, cooked and crumbled

2 large pickle spears, chopped

1 Place cream cheese in a large microwave-safe bowl and microwave for 45 seconds. Stir in mayonnaise, sour cream, onion, garlic powder, Worcestershire sauce, and 1 cup Cheddar. Add cooked ground beef and bacon. Sprinkle remaining Cheddar on top.

2 Place in 6" bowl and put into the air fryer basket.

3 Adjust the temperature to 400°F and set the timer for 10 minutes.

4 Dip is done when top is golden and bubbling. Sprinkle pickles over dish. Serve warm.

PER SERVING

CALORIES: 457	**FAT:** 35.0 g
PROTEIN: 21.6 g	**SODIUM:** 589 mg
FIBER: 0.2 g	**CARBOHYDRATES:** 3.8 g
NET CARBOHYDRATES: 3.6 g	**SUGAR:** 2.2 g

HOWEVER YOU LIKE IT!

Customize this dip with your favorite burger toppings! Caramelized onions and mushrooms, diced tomatoes, or jalapeños all make great additions! If you have a favorite burger sauce, try adding a drizzle to the top or mixing ¼ cup into the dip.

Pork Rind Tortillas

You won't believe how low-carb these Pork Rind Tortillas are! There's no need to buy low-carb tortillas at the store, which are usually made with wheat flour. With just a few simple ingredients, you'll have the perfect gluten-free base for tacos, burritos, or even chips!

- **Hands-On Time: 10 minutes**
- **Cook Time: 5 minutes**

Yields 4 tortillas (1 per serving)

1 ounce pork rinds

¾ cup shredded mozzarella cheese

2 tablespoons full-fat cream cheese

1 large egg

1 Place pork rinds into food processor and pulse until finely ground.

2 Place mozzarella into a large microwave-safe bowl. Break cream cheese into small pieces and add them to the bowl. Microwave for 30 seconds, or until both cheeses are melted and can easily be stirred together into a ball. Add ground pork rinds and egg to the cheese mixture.

3 Continue stirring until the mixture forms a ball. If it cools too much and cheese hardens, microwave for 10 more seconds.

4 Separate the dough into four small balls. Place each ball of dough between two sheets of parchment and roll into ¼" flat layer.

5 Place tortillas into the air fryer basket in single layer, working in batches if necessary.

6 Adjust the temperature to 400°F and set the timer for 5 minutes.

7 Tortillas will be crispy and firm when fully cooked. Serve immediately.

PER SERVING

CALORIES: 145	**FAT:** 10.0 g
PROTEIN: 10.7 g	**SODIUM:** 291 mg
FIBER: 0.0 g	**CARBOHYDRATES:** 0.8 g
NET CARBOHYDRATES: 0.8 g	**SUGAR:** 0.5 g

Mozzarella Sticks

Just like your restaurant favorites, these Mozzarella Sticks are covered in a crispy coating (but this coating is carb-free!) and full of gooey and delicious mozzarella. Pair this with your favorite low-carb marinara sauce, and dig right in! You can even customize it with your favorite kind of cheese for a different flavor profile.

- **Hands-On Time: 1 hour**
- **Cook Time: 10 minutes**

Yields 12 sticks (3 per serving)

6 (1-ounce) mozzarella string cheese sticks

½ cup grated Parmesan cheese

½ ounce pork rinds, finely ground

1 teaspoon dried parsley

2 large eggs

1 Place mozzarella sticks on a cutting board and cut in half. Freeze 45 minutes or until firm. If freezing overnight, remove frozen sticks after 1 hour and place into airtight zip-top storage bag and place back in freezer for future use.

2 In a large bowl, mix Parmesan, ground pork rinds, and parsley.

3 In a medium bowl, whisk eggs.

4 Dip a frozen mozzarella stick into beaten eggs and then into Parmesan mixture to coat. Repeat with remaining sticks. Place mozzarella sticks into the air fryer basket.

5 Adjust the temperature to 400°F and set the timer for 10 minutes or until golden.

6 Serve warm.

PER SERVING

CALORIES: 236	**FAT:** 13.8 g
PROTEIN: 19.2 g	**SODIUM:** 609 mg
FIBER: 0.0 g	**CARBOHYDRATES:** 4.7 g
NET CARBOHYDRATES: 4.7 g	**SUGAR:** 1.1 g

Bacon-Wrapped Onion Rings

These perfectly crispy onion rings can elevate your game day or take your juicy bunless burger to the next level. A medium onion has around 10 grams of carbs, which can seem high when you're limiting yourself to 20–50 grams of carbs per day. The zero-carb breading increases the fat and protein content for this appetizer, making it an even better keto option, as long as you enjoy in moderation.

- **Hands-On Time: 5 minutes**
- **Cook Time: 10 minutes**

Serves 4

1 large onion, peeled
1 tablespoon sriracha
8 slices sugar-free bacon

1 Slice onion into ¼"-thick slices. Brush sriracha over the onion slices. Take two slices of onion and wrap bacon around the rings. Repeat with remaining onion and bacon. Place into the air fryer basket.

2 Adjust the temperature to 350°F and set the timer for 10 minutes.

3 Use tongs to flip the onion rings halfway through the cooking time. When fully cooked, bacon will be crispy. Serve warm.

PER SERVING

CALORIES: 105	**FAT:** 5.9 g
PROTEIN: 7.5 g	**SODIUM:** 401 mg
FIBER: 0.6 g	**CARBOHYDRATES:** 4.3 g
NET CARBOHYDRATES: 3.7 g	**SUGAR:** 2.3 g

Mini Sweet Pepper Poppers

These crunchy bites are perfectly portioned, poppable peppers to please your palate. This bright and colorful twist on jalapeño poppers comes in bite-sized fun with bold flavor!

- **Hands-On Time: 15 minutes**
- **Cook Time: 8 minutes**

Yields 16 halves (4 per serving)

8 mini sweet peppers

4 ounces full-fat cream cheese, softened

4 slices sugar-free bacon, cooked and crumbled

¼ cup shredded pepper jack cheese

1 Remove the tops from the peppers and slice each one in half lengthwise. Use a small knife to remove seeds and membranes.

2 In a small bowl, mix cream cheese, bacon, and pepper jack.

3 Place 3 teaspoons of the mixture into each sweet pepper and press down smooth. Place into the fryer basket.

4 Adjust the temperature to 400°F and set the timer for 8 minutes.

5 Serve warm.

PER SERVING

CALORIES: 176	FAT: 13.4 g
PROTEIN: 7.4 g	SODIUM: 309 mg
FIBER: 0.9 g	CARBOHYDRATES: 3.6 g
NET CARBOHYDRATES: 2.7 g	SUGAR: 2.2 g

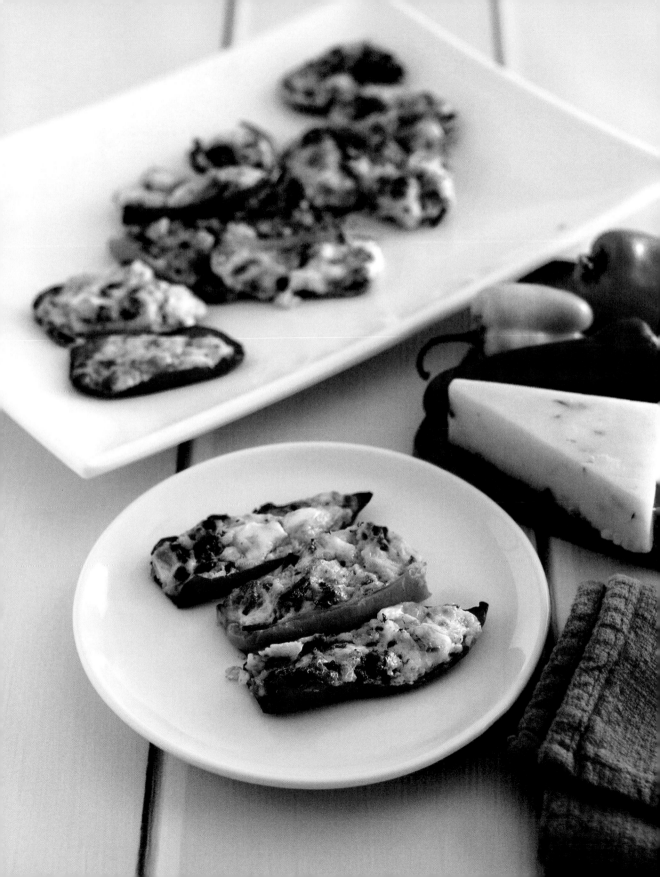

Spicy Spinach Artichoke Dip

This spicy twist on a classic appetizer pairs cool and creamy with jalapeños for the heavenly appetizer that every party needs! It's right at home on a platter of pork rinds or your favorite low-carb veggies, such as sliced cucumbers or celery sticks.

- **Hands-On Time: 10 minutes**
- **Cook Time: 10 minutes**

Serves 6

10 ounces frozen spinach, drained and thawed

1 (14-ounce) can artichoke hearts, drained and chopped

¼ cup chopped pickled jalapeños

8 ounces full-fat cream cheese, softened

¼ cup full-fat mayonnaise

¼ cup full-fat sour cream

½ teaspoon garlic powder

¼ cup grated Parmesan cheese

1 cup shredded pepper jack cheese

1 Mix all ingredients in a 4-cup baking bowl. Place into the air fryer basket.

2 Adjust the temperature to 320°F and set the timer for 10 minutes.

3 Remove when brown and bubbling. Serve warm.

PER SERVING

CALORIES: 226

PROTEIN: 10.0 g

FIBER: 3.7 g

NET CARBOHYDRATES: 6.5 g

FAT: 15.9 g

SODIUM: 776 mg

CARBOHYDRATES: 10.2 g

SUGAR: 3.4 g

Personal Mozzarella Pizza Crust

This pizza crust is nothing short of bread-like magic! Its applications are endless, and your air fryer can cook it and crisp it faster than your oven ever could! Top this crust with your favorite pizza toppings such as pepperoni, low-carb pizza sauce, and a sprinkle of cheese.

- **Hands-On Time: 5 minutes**
- **Cook Time: 10 minutes**

Serves 1

½ cup shredded whole-milk mozzarella cheese

2 tablespoons blanched finely ground almond flour

1 tablespoon full-fat cream cheese

1 large egg white

1 Place mozzarella, almond flour, and cream cheese in a medium microwave-safe bowl. Microwave for 30 seconds. Stir until smooth ball of dough forms. Add egg white and stir until soft round dough forms.

2 Press into a 6″ round pizza crust.

3 Cut a piece of parchment to fit your air fryer basket and place crust on parchment. Place into the air fryer basket.

4 Adjust the temperature to 350°F and set the timer for 10 minutes.

5 Flip after 5 minutes and at this time place any desired toppings on the crust. Continue cooking until golden. Serve immediately.

PER SERVING

CALORIES: 314	**FAT:** 22.7 g
PROTEIN: 19.9 g	**SODIUM:** 457 mg
FIBER: 1.5 g	**CARBOHYDRATES:** 5.1 g
NET CARBOHYDRATES: 3.6 g	**SUGAR:** 1.8 g

Garlic Cheese Bread

Who would've ever thought it would be so easy to satisfy your Garlic Cheese Bread cravings without an ounce of flour? Here's a keto-friendly appetizer that tastes just like delivery! Take it to the next level by dipping these strips in a low-carb marinara sauce!

- **Hands-On Time: 10 minutes**
- **Cook Time: 10 minutes**

Serves 2

1 cup shredded mozzarella cheese

¼ cup grated Parmesan cheese

1 large egg

½ teaspoon garlic powder

HIDDEN CARBS

Don't forget that cheese and eggs have carbs. Many nutrition labels round down if the amount is less than 1. An egg, for example, has 0.06 grams of carbs, even though it's often assumed to be carb-free.

1 Mix all ingredients in a large bowl. Cut a piece of parchment to fit your air fryer basket. Press the mixture into a circle on the parchment and place into the air fryer basket.

2 Adjust the temperature to 350°F and set the timer for 10 minutes.

3 Serve warm.

PER SERVING

CALORIES: 258	**FAT:** 16.6 g
PROTEIN: 19.2 g	**SODIUM:** 612 mg
FIBER: 0.1 g	**CARBOHYDRATES:** 3.7 g
NET CARBOHYDRATES: 3.6 g	**SUGAR:** 0.7 g

Crustless Three-Meat Pizza

Not all pizzas need a crust. And you can achieve crispy pizza perfection from scratch in minutes with this recipe. Even better, you can get creative with toppings to really make this pizza your own. Try topping with an Alfredo sauce and fresh veggies or a low-carb barbecue sauce and grilled chicken!

- **Hands-On Time: 5 minutes**
- **Cook Time: 5 minutes**

Serves 1

½ cup shredded mozzarella cheese

7 slices pepperoni

¼ cup cooked ground sausage

2 slices sugar-free bacon, cooked and crumbled

1 tablespoon grated Parmesan cheese

2 tablespoons low-carb, sugar-free pizza sauce, for dipping

1 Cover the bottom of a 6″ cake pan with mozzarella. Place pepperoni, sausage, and bacon on top of cheese and sprinkle with Parmesan. Place pan into the air fryer basket.

2 Adjust the temperature to 400°F and set the timer for 5 minutes.

3 Remove when cheese is bubbling and golden. Serve warm with pizza sauce for dipping.

PER SERVING

CALORIES: 466	FAT: 34.0 g
PROTEIN: 28.1 g	SODIUM: 1,446 mg
FIBER: 0.5 g	CARBOHYDRATES: 5.2 g
NET CARBOHYDRATES: 4.7 g	SUGAR: 1.6 g

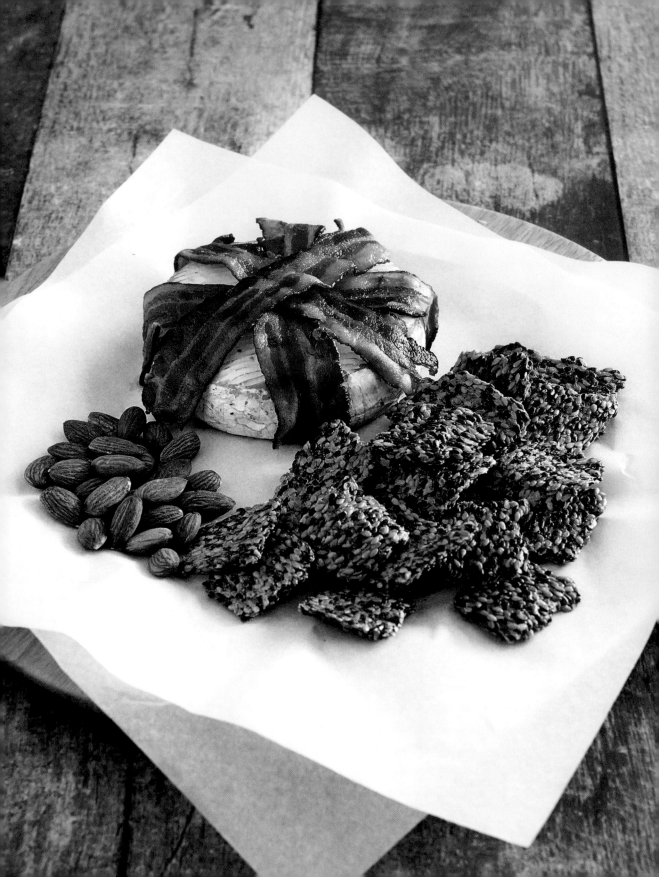

Bacon-Wrapped Brie

Many followers of the keto diet love to snack on cheese. That's because it has minimal carbs and is very convenient. Why not take it to the next level by wrapping the cheese in bacon? After you try this warm wheel of creamy cheese, you'll never want to go back to regular cheese!

- **Hands-On Time: 5 minutes**
- **Cook Time: 10 minutes**

Serves 8

4 slices sugar-free bacon
1 (8-ounce) round Brie

1 Place two slices of bacon to form an X. Place the third slice of bacon horizontally across the center of the X. Place the fourth slice of bacon vertically across the X. It should look like a plus sign (+) on top of an X. Place the Brie in the center of the bacon.

2 Wrap the bacon around the Brie, securing with a few toothpicks. Cut a piece of parchment to fit your air fryer basket and place the bacon-wrapped Brie on top. Place inside the air fryer basket.

3 Adjust the temperature to 400°F and set the timer for 10 minutes.

4 When 3 minutes remain on the timer, carefully flip Brie.

5 When cooked, bacon will be crispy and cheese will be soft and melty. To serve, cut into eight slices.

PER SERVING

CALORIES: 116	**FAT:** 8.9 g
PROTEIN: 7.7 g	**SODIUM:** 259 mg
FIBER: 0.0 g	**CARBOHYDRATES:** 0.2 g
NET CARBOHYDRATES: 0.2 g	**SUGAR:** 0.1 g

Smoky BBQ Roasted Almonds

As far as nuts go, almonds are a great low-carb option with plenty of healthy protein instead of carbs. A lot of flavored almonds you might find at your grocery store can be tasty but are usually processed with unnecessary ingredients, like maltodextrin, that can actually raise your blood sugar. This is a clean recipe for a flavorful snack any time of day!

- **Hands-On Time: 5 minutes**
- **Cook Time: 6 minutes**

Serves 4 (¼ cup per serving)

1 cup raw almonds
2 teaspoons coconut oil
1 teaspoon chili powder
¼ teaspoon cumin
¼ teaspoon smoked paprika
¼ teaspoon onion powder

1 In a large bowl, toss all ingredients until almonds are evenly coated with oil and spices. Place almonds into the air fryer basket.

2 Adjust the temperature to 320°F and set the timer for 6 minutes.

3 Toss the fryer basket halfway through the cooking time. Allow to cool completely.

PER SERVING

CALORIES: 182	**FAT:** 16.3 g
PROTEIN: 6.2 g	**SODIUM:** 19 mg
FIBER: 3.3 g	**CARBOHYDRATES:** 6.6 g
NET CARBOHYDRATES: 3.3 g	**SUGAR:** 1.1 g

HOMEMADE IS BETTER!
Store-bought barbecue-flavored almonds often have sugar as one of the first ingredients. It's best to avoid those because they add extra carbs. If you prefer more of a sweet barbecue flavor, try adding ½ teaspoon granular erythritol to your seasoning. The erythritol will caramelize a bit in the fryer and give your almonds a nice crunch.

Beef Jerky

It can be extremely difficult to find beef jerky that will work with your keto diet. Most brands you can find in the store are full of sugar or other ingredients that can spike your blood sugar and cause an insulin response, and most brands that are specifically low-carb can be very expensive with limited availability. With this recipe, you can have delicious jerky seasoned just the way you like!

- **Hands-On Time: 5 minutes**
- **Cook Time: 4 hours**

Serves 10

1 pound flat iron beef, thinly sliced
¼ cup soy sauce (or liquid aminos)
2 teaspoons Worcestershire sauce
¼ teaspoon crushed red pepper flakes
¼ teaspoon garlic powder
¼ teaspoon onion powder

1 Place all ingredients into a plastic storage bag or covered container and marinate 2 hours in refrigerator.

2 Place each slice of jerky on the air fryer rack in a single layer.

3 Adjust the temperature to 160°F and set the timer for 4 hours.

4 Cool and store in airtight container up to 1 week.

PER SERVING

CALORIES: 85
PROTEIN: 10.2 g
FIBER: 0.0 g
NET CARBOHYDRATES: 0.6 g

FAT: 3.5 g
SODIUM: 387 mg
CARBOHYDRATES: 0.6 g
SUGAR: 0.2 g

Pork Rind Nachos

Pork rinds are the ultimate replacement for chips. They're crunchy and flavorful, and best of all, they have zero carbs! Warm and gooey Pork Rind Nachos are a great snack for any time of day, and your air fryer will get the flavors just right!

- **Hands-On Time: 5 minutes**
- **Cook Time: 5 minutes**

Serves 2

1 ounce pork rinds

4 ounces shredded cooked chicken

½ cup shredded Monterey jack cheese

¼ cup sliced pickled jalapeños

¼ cup guacamole

¼ cup full-fat sour cream

1 Place pork rinds into 6" round baking pan. Cover with shredded chicken and Monterey jack cheese. Place pan into the air fryer basket.

2 Adjust the temperature to 370°F and set the timer for 5 minutes or until cheese is melted.

3 Top with jalapeños, guacamole, and sour cream. Serve immediately.

PER SERVING

CALORIES: 395

PROTEIN: 30.1 g

FIBER: 1.2 g

NET CARBOHYDRATES: 1.8 g

FAT: 27.5 g

SODIUM: 763 mg

CARBOHYDRATES: 3.0 g

SUGAR: 1.0 g

ALL PORK RINDS ARE NOT CREATED EQUAL

Pork rinds are an excellent low-carb chip replacement, but not all pork rinds are good quality. Many flavored pork rinds have added ingredients, such as sugars, and high glycemic binders such as maltodextrin, and some even have MSG! You may want to check out the health food section because sometimes it has better-quality pork rinds with cleaner ingredients.

Mozzarella-Stuffed Meatballs

The only thing better than juicy meatballs are juicy meatballs stuffed with gooey, melty cheese! You can enjoy this simple-to-season and easy-to-bake appetizer as is, or pump up the flavor by serving in a low-carb marinara sauce!

- **Hands-On Time: 15 minutes**
- **Cook Time: 15 minutes**

Yields 16 meatballs (4 per serving)

1 pound 80/20 ground beef
¼ cup blanched finely ground almond flour
1 teaspoon dried parsley
½ teaspoon garlic powder
¼ teaspoon onion powder
1 large egg
3 ounces low-moisture, whole-milk mozzarella, cubed
½ cup low-carb, no-sugar-added pasta sauce
¼ cup grated Parmesan cheese

INTERCHANGEABLE CHEESE!
You can customize this dish by swapping the mozzarella for your favorite cheese! For a taco-inspired meatball, add a packet of taco seasoning to your mix and use pepper jack or Cheddar cheese cubes for stuffing!

1 In a large bowl, add ground beef, almond flour, parsley, garlic powder, onion powder, and egg. Fold ingredients together until fully combined.

2 Form the mixture into 2″ balls and use your thumb or a spoon to create an indent in the center of each meatball. Place a cube of cheese in the center and form the ball around it.

3 Place the meatballs into the air fryer, working in batches if necessary.

4 Adjust the temperature to 350°F and set the timer for 15 minutes.

5 Meatballs will be slightly crispy on the outside and fully cooked when at least 180°F internally.

6 When they are finished cooking, toss the meatballs in the sauce and sprinkle with grated Parmesan for serving.

PER SERVING

CALORIES: 447	FAT: 29.7 g
PROTEIN: 29.6 g	SODIUM: 509 mg
FIBER: 1.8 g	CARBOHYDRATES: 5.4 g
NET CARBOHYDRATES: 3.6 g	SUGAR: 1.6 g

Ranch Roasted Almonds

Roasted almonds are low in carbs, but high in fiber and fats. They have a crunch that's hard to come by in low-carb foods and will satisfy your snacking urges. The only potential problem is their bland flavor, which this recipe eliminates completely!

- **Hands-On Time: 5 minutes**
- **Cook Time: 6 minutes**

Yields 2 cups (¹/₄ cup per serving)

2 cups raw almonds

2 tablespoons unsalted butter, melted

½ (1-ounce) ranch dressing mix packet

1 In a large bowl, toss almonds in butter to evenly coat. Sprinkle ranch mix over almonds and toss. Place almonds into the air fryer basket.

2 Adjust the temperature to 320°F and set the timer for 6 minutes.

3 Shake the basket two or three times during cooking.

4 Let cool at least 20 minutes. Almonds will be soft but become crunchier during cooling. Store in an airtight container up to 3 days.

PER SERVING

CALORIES: 190	**FAT:** 16.7 g
PROTEIN: 6.0 g	**SODIUM:** 133 mg
FIBER: 3.0 g	**CARBOHYDRATES:** 7.0 g
NET CARBOHYDRATES: 4.0 g	**SUGAR:** 1.0 g

4

Side Dishes

Side dishes can often be one of the most difficult foods to come up with to round out a keto-friendly meal. Traditional white rice or macaroni and cheese may be easy to throw together, but once you start your low-carb lifestyle, these dishes are no longer your friends. The carbs in many traditional side dishes can leave you feeling sluggish and will definitely prevent you from reaching ketosis. Thankfully, there are many delicious alternatives that your air fryer can help you prepare quickly and easily without ever needing to turn on your oven. This chapter will show you how to make recipes like Sausage-Stuffed Mushroom Caps and Cheesy Cauliflower Tots that will start a side dish revolution!

Loaded Roasted Broccoli

If you've ever thought broccoli was boring, this recipe will change your mind forever. It's stuffed to the gills with savory flavor and delicious fats to help keep you full, not to mention the great protein boost that comes from the broccoli itself!

- **Hands-On Time: 10 minutes**
- **Cook Time: 10 minutes**

Serves 2

3 cups fresh broccoli florets

1 tablespoon coconut oil

½ cup shredded sharp
   Cheddar cheese

¼ cup full-fat sour cream

4 slices sugar-free bacon,
   cooked and crumbled

1 scallion, sliced on the bias

1 Place broccoli into the air fryer basket and drizzle it with coconut oil.

2 Adjust the temperature to 350°F and set the timer for 10 minutes.

3 Toss the basket two or three times during cooking to avoid burned spots.

4 When broccoli begins to crisp at ends, remove from fryer. Top with shredded cheese, sour cream, and crumbled bacon and garnish with scallion slices.

PER SERVING

CALORIES: 361	FAT: 25.7 g
PROTEIN: 18.4 g	SODIUM: 564 mg
FIBER: 3.6 g	CARBOHYDRATES: 10.5 g
NET CARBOHYDRATES: 6.9 g	SUGAR: 3.3 g

Garlic Herb Butter Roasted Radishes

When roasted, radishes make a surprisingly excellent red potato substitute. When roasted in an air fryer, the crisp you're able to achieve is incomparable. Full of health benefits like vitamin C and healthy fiber, this is one side dish you'll always feel good about eating!

- **Hands-On Time: 10 minutes**
- **Cook Time: 10 minutes**

Serves 4

1 pound radishes

2 tablespoons unsalted butter, melted

½ teaspoon garlic powder

½ teaspoon dried parsley

¼ teaspoon dried oregano

¼ teaspoon ground black pepper

1 Remove roots from radishes and cut into quarters.

2 In a small bowl, add butter and seasonings. Toss the radishes in the herb butter and place into the air fryer basket.

3 Adjust the temperature to 350°F and set the timer for 10 minutes.

4 Halfway through the cooking time, toss the radishes in the air fryer basket. Continue cooking until edges begin to turn brown.

5 Serve warm.

PER SERVING

CALORIES: 63	FAT: 5.4 g
PROTEIN: 0.7 g	SODIUM: 28 mg
FIBER: 1.3 g	CARBOHYDRATES: 2.9 g
NET CARBOHYDRATES: 1.6 g	SUGAR: 1.4 g

Sausage-Stuffed Mushroom Caps

Mushrooms are very low-carb, are high in potassium, and have a fresh, earthy taste. Stuffing them with sausage boosts their protein and fat contents, and more importantly it elevates their flavor to something you won't be able to get enough of!

- **Hands-On Time: 10 minutes**
- **Cook Time: 8 minutes**

Serves 2

6 large portobello mushroom caps

½ pound Italian sausage

¼ cup chopped onion

2 tablespoons blanched finely ground almond flour

¼ cup grated Parmesan cheese

1 teaspoon minced fresh garlic

1 Use a spoon to hollow out each mushroom cap, reserving scrapings.

2 In a medium skillet over medium heat, brown the sausage about 10 minutes or until fully cooked and no pink remains. Drain and then add reserved mushroom scrapings, onion, almond flour, Parmesan, and garlic. Gently fold ingredients together and continue cooking an additional minute, then remove from heat.

3 Evenly spoon the mixture into mushroom caps and place the caps into a 6" round pan. Place pan into the air fryer basket.

4 Adjust the temperature to 375°F and set the timer for 8 minutes.

5 When finished cooking, the tops will be browned and bubbling. Serve warm.

PER SERVING

CALORIES: 404

PROTEIN: 24.3 g

FIBER: 4.5 g

NET CARBOHYDRATES: 13.7 g

FAT: 25.8 g

SODIUM: 1,106 mg

CARBOHYDRATES: 18.2 g

SUGAR: 8.1 g

Cheesy Cauliflower Tots

With the carb count in potatoes being so high, tater tots would be very difficult to fit into your macros. Luckily, cauliflower is a great substitute to give you that same crispy texture for a wonderfully kid-friendly side dish. Serve these warm with low-carb ketchup or your favorite dipping sauce.

- **Hands-On Time: 15 minutes**
- **Cook Time: 12 minutes**

Yields 16 tots (4 per serving)

1 large head cauliflower
1 cup shredded mozzarella cheese
½ cup grated Parmesan cheese
1 large egg
¼ teaspoon garlic powder
¼ teaspoon dried parsley
⅛ teaspoon onion powder

KID FRIENDLY!

These are great to make for kids because they look just like a classic tater tot, but they're much better for you. The cheese also helps to mask the cauliflower taste, making this the ultimate way to sneak veggies in!

1 On the stovetop, fill a large pot with 2 cups water and place a steamer in the pan. Bring water to a boil. Cut the cauliflower into florets and place on steamer basket. Cover pot with lid.

2 Allow cauliflower to steam 7 minutes until fork tender. Remove from steamer basket and place into cheesecloth or clean kitchen towel and let cool. Squeeze over sink to remove as much excess moisture as possible. The mixture will be too soft to form into tots if not all the moisture is removed. Mash with a fork to a smooth consistency.

3 Put the cauliflower into a large mixing bowl and add mozzarella, Parmesan, egg, garlic powder, parsley, and onion powder. Stir until fully combined. The mixture should be wet but easy to mold.

4 Take 2 tablespoons of the mixture and roll into tot shape. Repeat with remaining mixture. Place into the air fryer basket.

5 Adjust the temperature to 320°F and set the timer for 12 minutes.

6 Turn tots halfway through the cooking time. Cauliflower tots should be golden when fully cooked. Serve warm.

PER SERVING

CALORIES: 181	**FAT:** 9.5 g
PROTEIN: 13.5 g	**SODIUM:** 417 mg
FIBER: 3.0 g	**CARBOHYDRATES:** 9.6 g
NET CARBOHYDRATES: 6.6 g	**SUGAR:** 3.2 g

Crispy Brussels Sprouts

Get ready to cook some Brussels sprouts your kids will be excited about eating! They're rich in nutrients, including heart-healthy omega-3 fatty acids. This version is a complete reversal of the bland and boring Brussels sprouts you grew up eating!

- **Hands-On Time: 5 minutes**
- **Cook Time: 10 minutes**

Serves 4

1 pound Brussels sprouts
1 tablespoon coconut oil
1 tablespoon unsalted butter, melted

1 Remove all loose leaves from Brussels sprouts and cut each in half.

2 Drizzle sprouts with coconut oil and place into the air fryer basket.

3 Adjust the temperature to 400°F and set the timer for 10 minutes. You may want to gently stir halfway through the cooking time, depending on how they are beginning to brown.

4 When completely cooked, they should be tender with darker caramelized spots. Remove from fryer basket and drizzle with melted butter. Serve immediately.

PER SERVING

CALORIES: 90
PROTEIN: 2.9 g
FIBER: 3.2 g
NET CARBOHYDRATES: 4.3 g

FAT: 6.1 g
SODIUM: 21 mg
CARBOHYDRATES: 7.5 g
SUGAR: 1.9 g

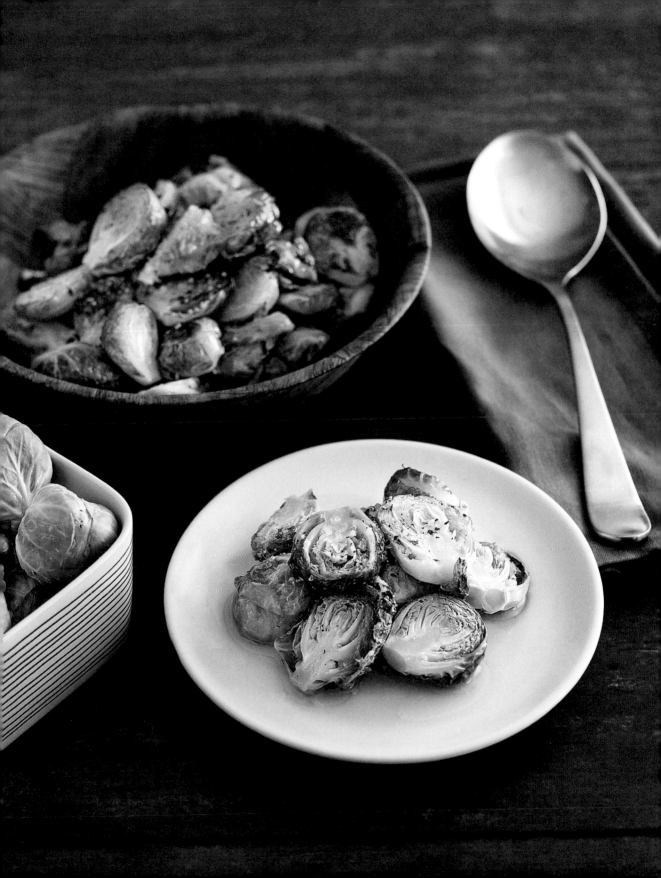

Zucchini Parmesan Chips

It can be difficult to get that satisfying crunch that a lot of carb-filled foods carry, but it's easier than ever with your air fryer. These thinly sliced zucchini chips are a nutrient-rich treat for mealtime or snack time!

- **Hands-On Time: 10 minutes**
- **Cook Time: 10 minutes**

Serves 4

2 medium zucchini
1 ounce pork rinds
½ cup grated Parmesan cheese
1 large egg

1 Slice zucchini in ¼"-thick slices. Place between two layers of paper towels or a clean kitchen towel for 30 minutes to remove excess moisture.

2 Place pork rinds into food processor and pulse until finely ground. Pour into medium bowl and mix with Parmesan.

3 Beat egg in a small bowl.

4 Dip zucchini slices in egg and then in pork rind mixture, coating as completely as possible. Carefully place each slice into the air fryer basket in a single layer, working in batches as necessary.

5 Adjust temperature to 320°F and set the timer for 10 minutes.

6 Flip chips halfway through the cooking time. Serve warm.

PER SERVING

CALORIES: 121	**FAT:** 6.7 g
PROTEIN: 9.9 g	**SODIUM:** 364 mg
FIBER: 0.6 g	**CARBOHYDRATES:** 3.8 g
NET CARBOHYDRATES: 3.2 g	**SUGAR:** 1.6 g

Roasted Garlic

Roasted garlic is one of the easiest ways to add a boost of flavor to any dish, from chicken to mashed cauliflower to the Roasted Garlic White Zucchini Rolls in Chapter 8. Unlike traditional oven recipes, which can take over an hour to get the roasted garlic right, your air fryer can extract all the savory flavor in just minutes!

- **Hands-On Time: 5 minutes**
- **Cook Time: 20 minutes**

Yields 12 cloves (1 per serving)

1 medium head garlic
2 teaspoons avocado oil

HOW TO USE ROASTED GARLIC

Roasted garlic has a milder, sweeter taste than raw garlic, which complements many dishes. Make a quick roasted garlic and herb butter for your steak or pork chops. Simply mash a clove of roasted garlic with ¼ cup softened butter and add your favorite herbs.

1 Remove any hanging excess peel from the garlic but leave the cloves covered. Cut off ¼ of the head of garlic, exposing the tips of the cloves.

2 Drizzle with avocado oil. Place the garlic head into a small sheet of aluminum foil, completely enclosing it. Place it into the air fryer basket.

3 Adjust the temperature to 400°F and set the timer for 20 minutes. If your garlic head is a bit smaller, check it after 15 minutes.

4 When done, garlic should be golden brown and very soft.

5 To serve, cloves should pop out and easily be spread or sliced. Store in an airtight container in the refrigerator up to 5 days. You may also freeze individual cloves on a baking sheet, then store together in a freezer-safe storage bag once frozen.

PER SERVING

CALORIES: 11	**FAT:** 0.7 g
PROTEIN: 0.2 g	**SODIUM:** 0 mg
FIBER: 0.1 g	**CARBOHYDRATES:** 1.0 g
NET CARBOHYDRATES: 0.9 g	**SUGAR:** 0.0 g

Kale Chips

With just the right seasoning and only a few minutes in your air fryer, you'll have a crispy snack that's easy to take on the go! Plus, kale is high in fiber, helping to promote a regular and healthy digestive tract.

- **Hands-On Time: 5 minutes**
- **Cook Time: 5 minutes**

Serves 4

4 cups stemmed kale
2 teaspoons avocado oil
½ teaspoon salt

1 In a large bowl, toss kale in avocado oil and sprinkle with salt. Place into the air fryer basket.

2 Adjust the temperature to 400°F and set the timer for 5 minutes.

3 Kale will be crispy when done. Serve immediately.

PER SERVING

CALORIES: 25	**FAT:** 2.2 g
PROTEIN: 0.5 g	**SODIUM:** 295 mg
FIBER: 0.4 g	**CARBOHYDRATES:** 1.1 g
NET CARBOHYDRATES: 0.7 g	**SUGAR:** 0.3 g

Buffalo Cauliflower

Cauliflower steaks are a great vegetarian option that have nutrients and flavor. Roasting them with buffalo sauce gives you a light and spicy dish that is totally guilt-free! Serve with crumbled blue cheese or ranch dressing if you need to tone down the spice!

- **Hands-On Time: 5 minutes**
- **Cook Time: 5 minutes**

Serves 4

4 cups cauliflower florets
2 tablespoons salted butter, melted
½ (1-ounce) dry ranch seasoning packet
¼ cup buffalo sauce

1 In a large bowl, toss cauliflower with butter and dry ranch. Place into the air fryer basket.

2 Adjust the temperature to 400°F and set the timer for 5 minutes.

3 Shake the basket two or three times during cooking. When tender, remove cauliflower from fryer basket and toss in buffalo sauce. Serve warm.

PER SERVING

CALORIES: 87	**FAT:** 5.6 g
PROTEIN: 2.1 g	**SODIUM:** 803 mg
FIBER: 2.1 g	**CARBOHYDRATES:** 7.3 g
NET CARBOHYDRATES: 5.2 g	**SUGAR:** 2.1 g

Green Bean Casserole

This low-carb spin on a potluck favorite will be the newest addition to your holiday menu. You'll notice the dish is missing the cream of mushroom soup you might be used to, but don't worry; you'll get all the traditional flavor without all the unnecessary carbs!

- **Hands-On Time: 10 minutes**
- **Cook Time: 15 minutes**

Serves 4

4 tablespoons unsalted butter

¼ cup diced yellow onion

½ cup chopped white mushrooms

½ cup heavy whipping cream

1 ounce full-fat cream cheese

½ cup chicken broth

¼ teaspoon xanthan gum

1 pound fresh green beans, edges trimmed

½ ounce pork rinds, finely ground

ARE GREEN BEANS KETO-FRIENDLY?

Green beans are legumes, but that doesn't mean you can't enjoy them on a ketogenic diet. Traditionally keto excluded legumes, including peanuts. Nowadays, a more rounded approach is taken and as long as the carbs are low and fit your macros, generally you can enjoy them. There are 3.6 grams net carbs in a 1-cup serving of green beans, which makes them a great choice!

1 In a medium skillet over medium heat, melt the butter. Sauté the onion and mushrooms until they become soft and fragrant, about 3–5 minutes.

2 Add the heavy whipping cream, cream cheese, and broth to the pan. Whisk until smooth. Bring to a boil and then reduce to a simmer. Sprinkle the xanthan gum into the pan and remove from heat.

3 Chop the green beans into 2" pieces and place into a 4-cup round baking dish. Pour the sauce mixture over them and stir until coated. Top the dish with ground pork rinds. Place into the air fryer basket.

4 Adjust the temperature to 320°F and set the timer for 15 minutes.

5 Top will be golden and green beans fork tender when fully cooked. Serve warm.

PER SERVING

CALORIES: 267	**FAT:** 23.4 g
PROTEIN: 3.6 g	**SODIUM:** 161 mg
FIBER: 3.2 g	**CARBOHYDRATES:** 9.7 g
NET CARBOHYDRATES: 6.5 g	**SUGAR:** 5.1 g

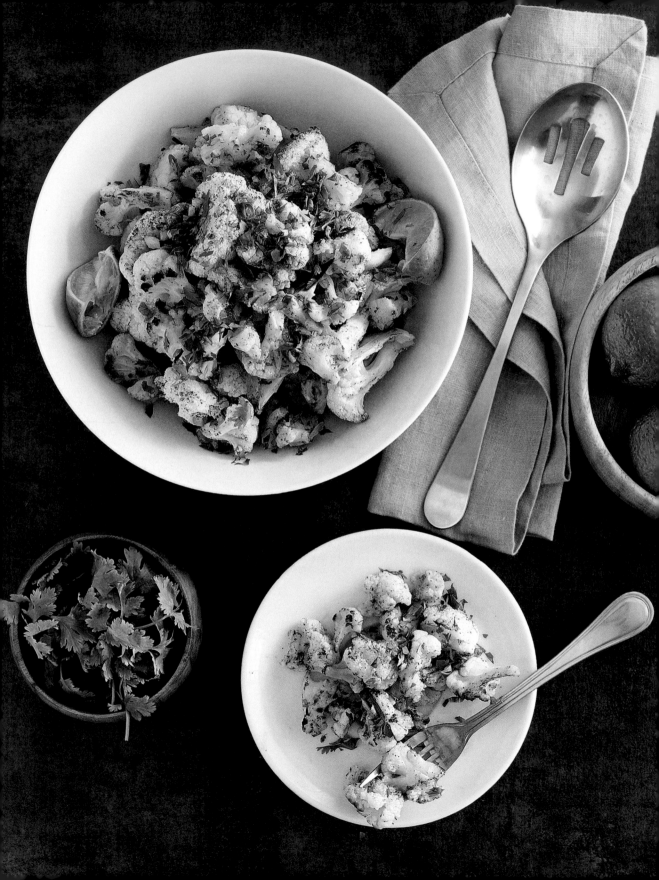

Cilantro Lime Roasted Cauliflower

Although it's rich in nutrients, like vitamin C, cauliflower is usually a pretty bland-tasting vegetable. This gives you an excellent opportunity to flavor it just the way you like for an appetizing side. This cilantro lime flavoring will complement any steak dish perfectly!

- **Hands-On Time: 10 minutes**
- **Cook Time: 7 minutes**

Serves 4

2 cups chopped cauliflower florets

2 tablespoons coconut oil, melted

2 teaspoons chili powder

½ teaspoon garlic powder

1 medium lime

2 tablespoons chopped cilantro

1 In a large bowl, toss cauliflower with coconut oil. Sprinkle with chili powder and garlic powder. Place seasoned cauliflower into the air fryer basket.

2 Adjust the temperature to 350°F and set the timer for 7 minutes.

3 Cauliflower will be tender and begin to turn golden at the edges. Place into serving bowl.

4 Cut the lime into quarters and squeeze juice over cauliflower. Garnish with cilantro.

PER SERVING

CALORIES: 73	**FAT:** 6.5 g
PROTEIN: 1.1 g	**SODIUM:** 16 mg
FIBER: 1.1 g	**CARBOHYDRATES:** 3.3 g
NET CARBOHYDRATES: 2.2 g	**SUGAR:** 1.1 g

Dinner Rolls

Do you miss bread on your keto diet? This low-carb substitute will satisfy any bread craving you may have and give you a great side dish to eat with your dinner. The dough can also be baked in a loaf pan or flattened out on a pizza pan to take care of you no matter which bread craving strikes!

- **Hands-On Time: 10 minutes**
- **Cook Time: 12 minutes**

Serves 6

1 cup shredded mozzarella cheese

1 ounce full-fat cream cheese

1 cup blanched finely ground almond flour

¼ cup ground flaxseed

½ teaspoon baking powder

1 large egg

1 Place mozzarella, cream cheese, and almond flour in a large microwave-safe bowl. Microwave for 1 minute. Mix until smooth.

2 Add flaxseed, baking powder, and egg until fully combined and smooth. Microwave an additional 15 seconds if it becomes too firm.

3 Separate the dough into six pieces and roll into balls. Place the balls into the air fryer basket.

4 Adjust the temperature to 320°F and set the timer for 12 minutes.

5 Allow rolls to cool completely before serving.

PER SERVING

CALORIES: 228	**FAT:** 18.1 g
PROTEIN: 10.8 g	**SODIUM:** 188 mg
FIBER: 3.9 g	**CARBOHYDRATES:** 6.8 g
NET CARBOHYDRATES: 2.9 g	**SUGAR:** 1.2 g

Coconut Flour Cheesy Garlic Biscuits

Missing biscuits on a keto diet is completely understandable. There's practically no dish they don't side perfectly with. Try these fluffy and flavorful treats with shrimp scampi for a keto-friendly at-home restaurant experience!

- **Hands-On Time: 10 minutes**
- **Cook Time: 12 minutes**

Serves 4

⅓ cup coconut flour
½ teaspoon baking powder
½ teaspoon garlic powder
1 large egg
¼ cup unsalted butter, melted and divided
½ cup shredded sharp Cheddar cheese
1 scallion, sliced

1 In a large bowl, mix coconut flour, baking powder, and garlic powder.

2 Stir in egg, half of the melted butter, Cheddar cheese, and scallions. Pour the mixture into a 6" round baking pan. Place into the air fryer basket.

3 Adjust the temperature to 320°F and set the timer for 12 minutes.

4 To serve, remove from pan and allow to fully cool. Slice into four pieces and pour remaining melted butter over each.

PER SERVING

CALORIES: 218	**FAT:** 16.9 g
PROTEIN: 7.2 g	**SODIUM:** 177 mg
FIBER: 3.4 g	**CARBOHYDRATES:** 6.8 g
NET CARBOHYDRATES: 3.4 g	**SUGAR:** 2.1 g

Radish Chips

Radishes might not come to mind right away when thinking about healthy, low-carb vegetables, but this recipe might just change that forever. This quick and healthy snack packs plenty of flavor as well as dietary fiber to help you feel full and avoid overeating.

- **Hands-On Time: 10 minutes**
- **Cook Time: 5 minutes**

Serves 4

2 cups water
1 pound radishes
¼ teaspoon onion powder
¼ teaspoon paprika
½ teaspoon garlic powder
2 tablespoons coconut oil, melted

1 Place water in a medium saucepan and bring to a boil on stovetop.

2 Remove the top and bottom from each radish, then use a mandoline to slice each radish thin and uniformly. You may also use the slicing blade in the food processor for this step.

3 Place the radish slices into the boiling water for 5 minutes or until translucent. Remove them from the water and place them into a clean kitchen towel to absorb excess moisture.

4 Toss the radish chips in a large bowl with remaining ingredients until fully coated in oil and seasoning. Place radish chips into the air fryer basket.

5 Adjust the temperature to 320°F and set the timer for 5 minutes.

6 Shake the basket two or three times during the cooking time. Serve warm.

PER SERVING

CALORIES: 77	**FAT:** 6.5 g
PROTEIN: 0.8 g	**SODIUM:** 40 mg
FIBER: 1.8 g	**CARBOHYDRATES:** 4.0 g
NET CARBOHYDRATES: 2.2 g	**SUGAR:** 2.0 g

Flatbread

Flatbread is a great alternative for anything from a tortilla to a pizza crust. This easy recipe is flexible and versatile so you can make it any time of day to make your meal more filling.

- **Hands-On Time: 5 minutes**
- **Cook Time: 7 minutes**

Serves 2

1 cup shredded mozzarella cheese

¼ cup blanched finely ground almond flour

1 ounce full-fat cream cheese, softened

1 In a large microwave-safe bowl, melt mozzarella in the microwave for 30 seconds. Stir in almond flour until smooth and then add cream cheese. Continue mixing until dough forms, gently kneading it with wet hands if necessary.

2 Divide the dough into two pieces and roll out to ¼" thickness between two pieces of parchment. Cut another piece of parchment to fit your air fryer basket.

3 Place a piece of flatbread onto your parchment and into the air fryer, working in two batches if needed.

4 Adjust the temperature to 320°F and set the timer for 7 minutes.

5 Halfway through the cooking time flip the flatbread. Serve warm.

PER SERVING

CALORIES: 296	FAT: 22.6 g
PROTEIN: 16.3 g	SODIUM: 402 mg
FIBER: 1.5 g	CARBOHYDRATES: 4.8 g
NET CARBOHYDRATES: 3.3 g	SUGAR: 1.5 g

Avocado Fries

Avocados are an absolute staple on the keto diet. That's because they're low in carbs and very high in healthy fats that keep you full and focused. Some people like to eat avocados plain, but if you're not one of them, try these crispy Avocado Fries; they are a great, easy way to boost an avocado's flavor with little effort!

- **Hands-On Time: 15 minutes**
- **Cook Time: 5 minutes**

Serves 4

2 medium avocados
1 ounce pork rinds, finely ground

1 Cut each avocado in half. Remove the pit. Carefully remove the peel and then slice the flesh into ¼"-thick slices.

2 Place the pork rinds into a medium bowl and press each piece of avocado into the pork rinds to coat completely. Place the avocado pieces into the air fryer basket.

3 Adjust the temperature to 350°F and set the timer for 5 minutes.

4 Serve immediately.

PER SERVING

CALORIES: 153	**FAT:** 11.9 g
PROTEIN: 5.4 g	**SODIUM:** 121 mg
FIBER: 4.6 g	**CARBOHYDRATES:** 5.9 g
NET CARBOHYDRATES: 1.3 g	**SUGAR:** 0.2 g

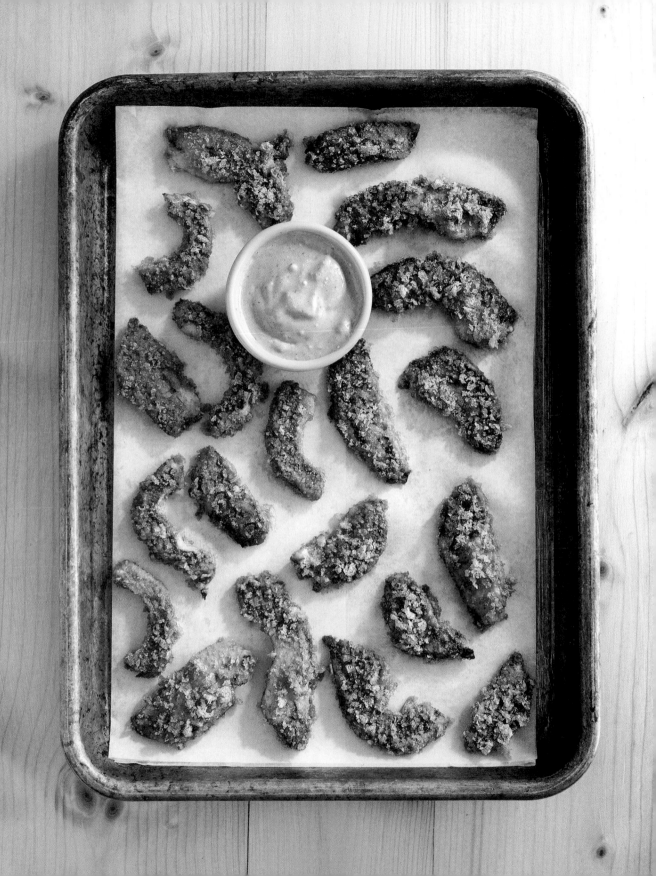

Pita-Style Chips

You'll never miss the real thing with these chips! They come out amazingly crunchy and perfect for dipping! Try them with the Bacon Cheeseburger Dip (Chapter 3) or add some Mexican-style toppings for yummy nachos!

- **Hands-On Time: 10 minutes**
- **Cook Time: 5 minutes**

Serves 4

1 cup shredded mozzarella cheese

½ ounce pork rinds, finely ground

¼ cup blanched finely ground almond flour

1 large egg

1 Place mozzarella in a large microwave-safe bowl and microwave for 30 seconds or until melted. Add remaining ingredients and stir until a mostly smooth dough forms into a ball easily. If dough is too hard, microwave for 15 seconds.

2 Roll dough out between two pieces of parchment into a large rectangle and then use a knife to cut triangle shaped chips. Place the chips into the air fryer basket.

3 Adjust the temperature to 350°F and set the timer for 5 minutes.

4 Chips will be golden in color and firm when done. As they cool, they will become even more firm.

PER SERVING

CALORIES: 161

PROTEIN: 11.3 g

FIBER: 0.8 g

NET CARBOHYDRATES: 1.4 g

FAT: 11.6 g

SODIUM: 251 mg

CARBOHYDRATES: 2.2 g

SUGAR: 0.6 g

Roasted Eggplant

Eggplant is a very low-calorie vegetable that is high in fiber. This combination can be great for promoting weight loss, and luckily eggplant is very easy to add to your diet. This simple roasting method makes for a tasty side that would go great with other veggies or a yummy chicken dish.

- **Hands-On Time: 15 minutes**
- **Cook Time: 15 minutes**

Serves 4

1 large eggplant
2 tablespoons olive oil
¼ teaspoon salt
½ teaspoon garlic powder

1 Remove top and bottom from eggplant. Slice eggplant into ¼"-thick round slices.

2 Brush slices with olive oil. Sprinkle with salt and garlic powder. Place eggplant slices into the air fryer basket.

3 Adjust the temperature to 390°F and set the timer for 15 minutes.

4 Serve immediately.

PER SERVING

CALORIES: 91
PROTEIN: 1.3 g
FIBER: 3.7 g
NET CARBOHYDRATES: 3.8 g

FAT: 6.7 g
SODIUM: 147 mg
CARBOHYDRATES: 7.5 g
SUGAR: 4.4 g

Parmesan Herb Focaccia Bread

This herb-baked focaccia substitute has only a fraction of carbs as the real thing, but it's the perfect sandwich bread to make sure you never feel left out while living your low-carb lifestyle.

- **Hands-On Time: 10 minutes**
- **Cook Time: 10 minutes**

Serves 6

1 cup shredded mozzarella cheese

1 ounce full-fat cream cheese

1 cup blanched finely ground almond flour

¼ cup ground golden flaxseed

¼ cup grated Parmesan cheese

½ teaspoon baking soda

2 large eggs

½ teaspoon garlic powder

¼ teaspoon dried basil

¼ teaspoon dried rosemary

2 tablespoons salted butter, melted and divided

SANDWICHES ARE BACK ON THE MENU!

For a filling meal, you can allow the bread to fully cool, then slice the entire round in half. Make it a club sandwich with turkey, bacon, lettuce, tomato, and mayo, or whatever your favorite toppings may be. Replace the top and slice into six pieces to serve. It's an easy meal for the whole family!

1 Place mozzarella, cream cheese, and almond flour into a large microwave-safe bowl and microwave for 1 minute. Add the flaxseed, Parmesan, and baking soda and stir until smooth ball forms. If the mixture cools too much, it will be hard to mix. Return to microwave for 10–15 seconds to rewarm if necessary.

2 Stir in eggs. You may need to use your hands to get them fully incorporated. Just keep stirring and they will absorb into the dough.

3 Sprinkle dough with garlic powder, basil, and rosemary and knead into dough. Grease a 6" round baking pan with 1 tablespoon melted butter. Press the dough evenly into the pan. Place pan into the air fryer basket.

4 Adjust the temperature to 400°F and set the timer for 10 minutes.

5 At 7 minutes, cover with foil if bread begins to get too dark.

6 Remove and let cool at least 30 minutes. Drizzle with remaining butter and serve.

PER SERVING

CALORIES: 292	**FAT:** 23.4 g
PROTEIN: 13.1 g	**SODIUM:** 370 mg
FIBER: 4.0 g	**CARBOHYDRATES:** 7.6 g
NET CARBOHYDRATES: 3.6 g	**SUGAR:** 1.2 g

Quick and Easy Home Fries

Jicama may seem like an intimidating vegetable from the outside but it's very easy to work with and well worth the extra effort. Peeling a jicama is a bit tricky but using a sharp knife to slice the peel off works easily. If you've never tasted it before, it's similar to a white potato in texture but with a hint of sweetness. It absorbs flavors easily, which makes jicama a good potato substitute. For a fraction of the carbs of the original, these home fries are the perfect smart swap for your keto diet.

- **Hands-On Time: 10 minutes**
- **Cook Time: 10 minutes**

Serves 4

1 medium jicama, peeled

1 tablespoon coconut oil, melted

¼ teaspoon ground black pepper

½ teaspoon pink Himalayan salt

1 medium green bell pepper, seeded and diced

½ medium white onion, peeled and diced

1 Cut jicama into 1" cubes. Place into a large bowl and toss with coconut oil until coated. Sprinkle with pepper and salt. Place into the air fryer basket with peppers and onion.

2 Adjust the temperature to 400°F and set the timer for 10 minutes.

3 Shake two or three times during cooking. Jicama will be tender and dark around edges. Serve immediately.

PER SERVING

CALORIES: 97	FAT: 3.3 g
PROTEIN: 1.5 g	SODIUM: 202 mg
FIBER: 8.0 g	CARBOHYDRATES: 15.8 g
NET CARBOHYDRATES: 7.8 g	SUGAR: 4.0 g

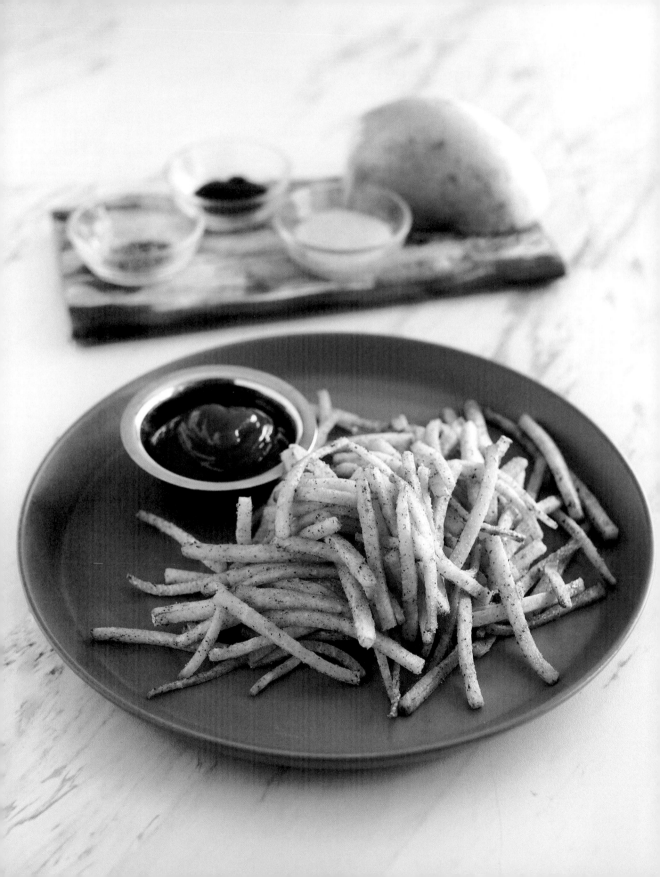

Jicama Fries

Jicama, also known as a *Mexican potato*, is a root vegetable native to Central and South America. A jicama is loaded with fiber, and it makes an excellent replacement for traditional French fries! One major selling point of air fryers is that they can get your French fries extremely crispy, with little to no oil. With this recipe you can take part in the fun, in a way that's much better for you!

- **Hands-On Time: 10 minutes**
- **Cook Time: 20 minutes**

Serves 4

1 small jicama, peeled
¾ teaspoon chili powder
¼ teaspoon garlic powder
¼ teaspoon onion powder
¼ teaspoon ground black pepper

WHERE CAN YOU FIND JICAMA?

Jicama is more common to grocery stores than you might realize! Check your produce aisle near regular potatoes, but if your search is unsuccessful be sure to try an international market.

1 Cut jicama into matchstick-sized pieces.

2 Place pieces into a small bowl and sprinkle with remaining ingredients. Place the fries into the air fryer basket.

3 Adjust the temperature to 350°F and set the timer for 20 minutes.

4 Toss the basket two or three times during cooking. Serve warm.

PER SERVING

CALORIES: 37	FAT: 0.1 g
PROTEIN: 0.8 g	SODIUM: 18 mg
FIBER: 4.7 g	CARBOHYDRATES: 8.7 g
NET CARBOHYDRATES: 4.0 g	SUGAR: 1.7 g

Fried Green Tomatoes

Green tomatoes are tomatoes that haven't fully ripened. Because of this, they're tarter than a red tomato and firmer. Fried Green Tomatoes are a sweet and juicy side that taste like summer with every bite and come together easily in your air fryer, so you don't have to worry about frying them in oil!

- **Hands-On Time: 10 minutes**
- **Cook Time: 7 minutes**

Serves 4

2 medium green tomatoes

1 large egg

¼ cup blanched finely ground almond flour

⅓ cup grated Parmesan cheese

1 Slice tomatoes into ½"-thick slices. In a medium bowl, whisk the egg. In a large bowl, mix the almond flour and Parmesan.

2 Dip each tomato slice into the egg, then dredge in the almond flour mixture. Place the slices into the air fryer basket.

3 Adjust the temperature to 400°F and set the timer for 7 minutes.

4 Flip the slices halfway through the cooking time. Serve immediately.

PER SERVING

CALORIES: 106	FAT: 6.7 g
PROTEIN: 6.2 g	SODIUM: 175 mg
FIBER: 1.4 g	CARBOHYDRATES: 5.9 g
NET CARBOHYDRATES: 4.5 g	SUGAR: 2.8 g

Fried Pickles

A favorite for many people in the Southern United States, Fried Pickles are a crispy and tart appetizer. They're traditionally battered with cornmeal and flour, but this keto-friendly alternative will give you all the flavor you need. Pair them with Southern "Fried" Chicken (Chapter 5) to keep the authentic Southern feel going!

- **Hands-On Time: 10 minutes**
- **Cook Time: 5 minutes**

Serves 4

1 tablespoon coconut flour
⅓ cup blanched finely ground
   almond flour
1 teaspoon chili powder
¼ teaspoon garlic powder
1 large egg
1 cup sliced pickles

1 Whisk coconut flour, almond flour, chili powder, and garlic powder together in a medium bowl.

2 Whisk egg in a small bowl.

3 Pat each pickle with a paper towel and dip into the egg. Then dredge in the flour mixture. Place pickles into the air fryer basket.

4 Adjust the temperature to 400°F and set the timer for 5 minutes.

5 Flip the pickles halfway through the cooking time.

PER SERVING

CALORIES: 85	**FAT:** 6.1 g
PROTEIN: 4.3 g	**SODIUM:** 351 mg
FIBER: 2.3 g	**CARBOHYDRATES:** 4.6 g
NET CARBOHYDRATES: 2.3 g	**SUGAR:** 1.2 g

5

Chicken Main Dishes

Chicken is probably already one of the most commonly eaten meats in your household. It's hard to compete with its affordability and convenience, plus chicken is an excellent source of protein, and it can be a great source of fat too! The problem? Chicken can get a little boring. Luckily, this chapter is full of healthy and exciting ideas that will bring a whole new light to dinnertime. From Crispy Buffalo Chicken Tenders to Chicken Pizza Crust, you'll have no shortage of amazing meals to add to your weekly rotation!

Crispy Buffalo Chicken Tenders

Your days of delicious crispy chicken aren't over just because you don't eat traditional breading! This recipe replaces the carb-filled, heavy wheat flour or bread crumbs you might be used to with an amazing zero-carb substitute: pork rinds! Serve these with ranch dressing or your favorite dipping sauce.

- **Hands-On Time: 15 minutes**
- **Cook Time: 20 minutes**

Serves 4

1 pound boneless, skinless chicken tenders
¼ cup hot sauce
1½ ounces pork rinds, finely ground
1 teaspoon chili powder
1 teaspoon garlic powder

1 Place chicken tenders in large bowl and pour hot sauce over them. Toss tenders in hot sauce, evenly coating.

2 In a separate large bowl, mix ground pork rinds with chili powder and garlic powder.

3 Place each tender in the ground pork rinds, covering completely. Wet your hands with water and press down the pork rinds into the chicken.

4 Place the tenders in a single layer into the air fryer basket.

5 Adjust the temperature to 375°F and set the timer for 20 minutes.

6 Serve warm.

PER SERVING

CALORIES: 160	**FAT:** 4.4 g
PROTEIN: 27.3 g	**SODIUM:** 387 mg
FIBER: 0.4 g	**CARBOHYDRATES:** 1.0 g
NET CARBOHYDRATES: 0.6 g	**SUGAR:** 0.1 g

Teriyaki Wings

These marinated wings are dripping with finger-licking flavor and are supereasy to prepare! The garlic and ginger give this recipe a bit of a kick while the teriyaki sauce adds some salt to bring out the wings' natural flavors. Before air frying, you toss the wings in baking powder for extra crispy skin rivaling traditional breaded wings!

- **Hands-On Time: 1 hour**
- **Cook Time: 25 minutes**

Serves 4

2 pounds chicken wings
½ cup sugar-free teriyaki
    sauce
2 teaspoons minced garlic
¼ teaspoon ground ginger
2 teaspoons baking powder

1 Place all ingredients except baking powder into a large bowl or bag and let marinade for 1 hour in the refrigerator.

2 Place wings into the air fryer basket and sprinkle with baking powder. Gently rub into wings.

3 Adjust the temperature to 400°F and set the timer for 25 minutes.

4 Toss the basket two or three times during cooking.

5 Wings should be crispy and cooked to at least 165°F internally when done. Serve immediately.

PER SERVING

CALORIES: 446	FAT: 29.8 g
PROTEIN: 41.8 g	SODIUM: 1,034 mg
FIBER: 0.1 g	CARBOHYDRATES: 3.2 g
NET CARBOHYDRATES: 3.1 g	SUGAR: 0.0 g

Lemon Thyme Roasted Chicken

Who knew you could perfectly roast an entire chicken in your air fryer? In less time, and with more even convection cooking than a standard oven, it'll be tough to go back to your old way!

- **Hands-On Time: 10 minutes**
- **Cook Time: 60 minutes**

Serves 6

1 (4-pound) chicken
2 teaspoons dried thyme
1 teaspoon garlic powder
½ teaspoon onion powder
2 teaspoons dried parsley
1 teaspoon baking powder
1 medium lemon
2 tablespoons salted butter, melted

AIR FRYER SIZE MATTERS

Depending on your air fryer size, you may be able to cook a larger chicken. Some air fryers can fit a 6-pound chicken whereas smaller ones may not be able to. If you have a smaller air fryer, you can also try cutting the chicken in half at the backbone and cooking it in two batches.

1 Rub chicken with thyme, garlic powder, onion powder, parsley, and baking powder.

2 Slice lemon and place four slices on top of chicken, breast side up, and secure with toothpicks. Place remaining slices inside of the chicken.

3 Place entire chicken into the air fryer basket, breast side down.

4 Adjust the temperature to 350°F and set the timer for 60 minutes.

5 After 30 minutes, flip chicken so breast side is up.

6 When done, internal temperature should be 165°F and the skin golden and crispy. To serve, pour melted butter over entire chicken.

PER SERVING

CALORIES: 504	**FAT:** 36.8 g
PROTEIN: 32.0 g	**SODIUM:** 240 mg
FIBER: 0.3 g	**CARBOHYDRATES:** 1.4 g
NET CARBOHYDRATES: 1.1 g	**SUGAR:** 0.2 g

Cilantro Lime Chicken Thighs

Chicken thighs are a more affordable and fattier cut of chicken compared to chicken breasts—perfect for anyone following the keto diet! Along with the fat comes succulent flavor bursting through the skin. Paired with cilantro lime seasoning, this recipe is perfection.

- **Hands-On Time: 15 minutes**
- **Cook Time: 22 minutes**

Serves 4

4 bone-in, skin-on chicken thighs
1 teaspoon baking powder
½ teaspoon garlic powder
2 teaspoons chili powder
1 teaspoon cumin
2 medium limes
¼ cup chopped fresh cilantro

A CUT ABOVE THE REST!

Chicken thighs have much more fat than chicken breasts, which makes them perfect for the keto diet. They can seem intimidating if you aren't used to cooking them, but they're packed with flavor and worth the extra effort. For added flavor, pull up the skin on one side and stuff some seasoning in it so the meat is flavored, not just the skin.

1 Pat chicken thighs dry and sprinkle with baking powder.

2 In a small bowl, mix garlic powder, chili powder, and cumin and sprinkle evenly over thighs, gently rubbing on and under chicken skin.

3 Cut one lime in half and squeeze juice over thighs. Place chicken into the air fryer basket.

4 Adjust the temperature to 380°F and set the timer for 22 minutes.

5 Cut other lime into four wedges for serving and garnish cooked chicken with wedges and cilantro.

PER SERVING

CALORIES: 435	**FAT:** 29.1 g
PROTEIN: 32.3 g	**SODIUM:** 317 mg
FIBER: 0.6 g	**CARBOHYDRATES:** 2.6 g
NET CARBOHYDRATES: 2.0 g	**SUGAR:** 0.3 g

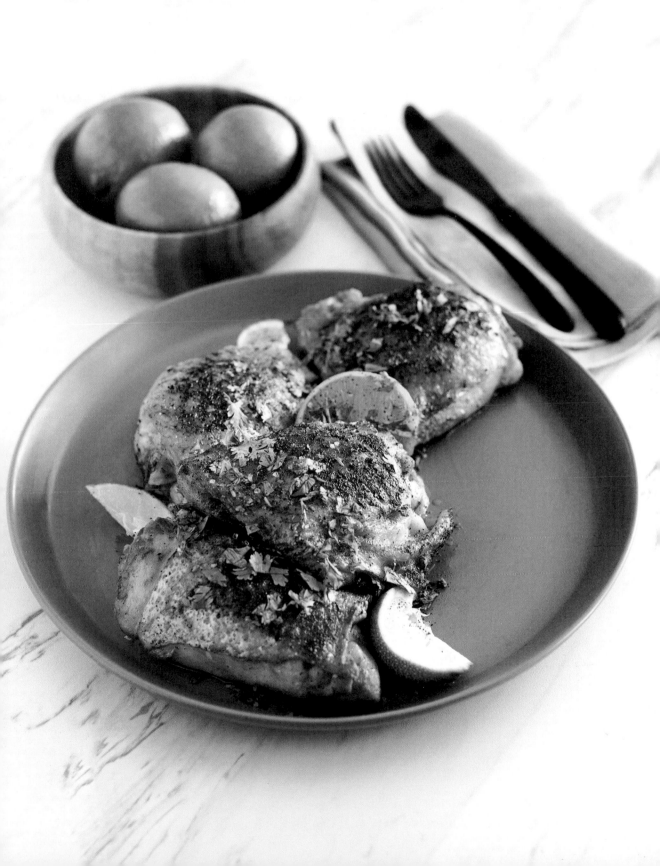

Lemon Pepper Drumsticks

Lemon pepper is a popular coating for keto-friendly chicken because it's a simple, savory, dry-rub seasoning with no reason to add unnecessary carbs. When you crisp these drumsticks in your air fryer, that seasoning soaks into the chicken skin, giving each bite a zesty flair!

- **Hands-On Time: 5 minutes**
- **Cook Time: 25 minutes**

Yields 8 drumsticks (2 per serving)

2 teaspoons baking powder
½ teaspoon garlic powder
8 chicken drumsticks
4 tablespoons salted butter, melted
1 tablespoon lemon pepper seasoning

1 Sprinkle baking powder and garlic powder over drumsticks and rub into chicken skin. Place drumsticks into the air fryer basket.

2 Adjust the temperature to 375°F and set the timer for 25 minutes.

3 Use tongs to turn drumsticks halfway through the cooking time.

4 When skin is golden and internal temperature is at least 165°F, remove from fryer.

5 In a large bowl, mix butter and lemon pepper seasoning. Add drumsticks to the bowl and toss until coated. Serve warm.

PER SERVING

CALORIES: 532	FAT: 32.3 g
PROTEIN: 48.3 g	SODIUM: 706 mg
FIBER: 0.0 g	CARBOHYDRATES: 1.2 g
NET CARBOHYDRATES: 1.2 g	SUGAR: 0.0 g

Fajita-Stuffed Chicken Breast

This dish is so good you won't even miss the tortilla! The smoky spices create a flavorful crust on the chicken while the veggies brighten up your meal. For a cheesy twist, sprinkle a half cup of shredded Monterey jack cheese on top of the chicken rolls before baking.

- **Hands-On Time: 15 minutes**
- **Cook Time: 25 minutes**

Serves 4

2 (6-ounce) boneless, skinless chicken breasts

¼ medium white onion, peeled and sliced

1 medium green bell pepper, seeded and sliced

1 tablespoon coconut oil

2 teaspoons chili powder

1 teaspoon ground cumin

½ teaspoon garlic powder

1 Slice each chicken breast completely in half lengthwise into two even pieces. Using a meat tenderizer, pound out the chicken until it's about ¼" thickness.

2 Lay each slice of chicken out and place three slices of onion and four slices of green pepper on the end closest to you. Begin rolling the peppers and onions tightly into the chicken. Secure the roll with either toothpicks or a couple pieces of butcher's twine.

3 Drizzle coconut oil over chicken. Sprinkle each side with chili powder, cumin, and garlic powder. Place each roll into the air fryer basket.

4 Adjust the temperature to 350°F and set the timer for 25 minutes.

5 Serve warm.

PER SERVING

CALORIES: 146	**FAT:** 4.9 g
PROTEIN: 19.8 g	**SODIUM:** 78 mg
FIBER: 1.2 g	**CARBOHYDRATES:** 3.2 g
NET CARBOHYDRATES: 2.0 g	**SUGAR:** 1.1 g

Chicken Parmesan

Chicken Parmesan is a popular Italian dish that is usually made with breaded chicken covered in tomato sauce and cheese, served over spaghetti. This recipe cuts not only the carbs from the breading but also the unnecessary sugar that is used in most tomato sauces.

- **Hands-On Time: 10 minutes**
- **Cook Time: 25 minutes**

Serves 4

2 (6-ounce) boneless, skinless chicken breasts

½ teaspoon garlic powder

¼ teaspoon dried oregano

½ teaspoon dried parsley

4 tablespoons full-fat mayonnaise, divided

1 cup shredded mozzarella cheese, divided

1 ounce pork rinds, crushed

½ cup grated Parmesan cheese, divided

1 cup low-carb, no-sugar-added pasta sauce

MAKE IT A MEAL!
Serve this Chicken Parmesan over zucchini noodles or spaghetti squash to round out the dish. Don't forget to top it with some fresh grated Parmesan!

1 Slice each chicken breast in half lengthwise and pound out to ¾" thickness. Sprinkle with garlic powder, oregano, and parsley.

2 Spread 1 tablespoon mayonnaise on top of each piece of chicken, then sprinkle ¼ cup mozzarella on each piece.

3 In a small bowl, mix the crushed pork rinds and Parmesan. Sprinkle the mixture on top of mozzarella.

4 Pour sauce into 6" round baking pan and place chicken on top. Place pan into the air fryer basket.

5 Adjust the temperature to 320°F and set the timer for 25 minutes.

6 Cheese will be browned and internal temperature of the chicken will be at least 165°F when fully cooked. Serve warm.

PER SERVING

CALORIES: 393	**FAT:** 22.8 g
PROTEIN: 34.2 g	**SODIUM:** 983 mg
FIBER: 2.1 g	**CARBOHYDRATES:** 6.8 g
NET CARBOHYDRATES: 4.7 g	**SUGAR:** 2.4 g

Chicken Cordon Bleu Casserole

This ultra creamy casserole gives you all the flavors of traditional cordon bleu without the carbs! Crushed pork rinds give this dish a crunchy topping. Don't worry if you aren't a fan of pork rinds; you can use crushed pure cheese crisps! Just be sure there's no added flours in the crisps.

- **Hands-On Time: 15 minutes**
- **Cook Time: 15 minutes**

Serves 4

2 cups cubed cooked chicken thigh meat

½ cup cubed cooked ham

2 ounces Swiss cheese, cubed

4 ounces full-fat cream cheese, softened

1 tablespoon heavy cream

2 tablespoons unsalted butter, melted

2 teaspoons Dijon mustard

1 ounce pork rinds, crushed

1 Place chicken and ham into a 6" round baking pan and toss so meat is evenly mixed. Sprinkle cheese cubes on top of meat.

2 In a large bowl, mix cream cheese, heavy cream, butter, and mustard and then pour the mixture over the meat and cheese. Top with pork rinds. Place pan into the air fryer basket.

3 Adjust the temperature to 350°F and set the timer for 15 minutes.

4 The casserole will be browned and bubbling when done. Serve warm.

PER SERVING

CALORIES: 403	**FAT:** 28.2 g
PROTEIN: 30.7 g	**SODIUM:** 660 mg
FIBER: 0.0 g	**CARBOHYDRATES:** 2.3 g
NET CARBOHYDRATES: 2.3 g	**SUGAR:** 1.2 g

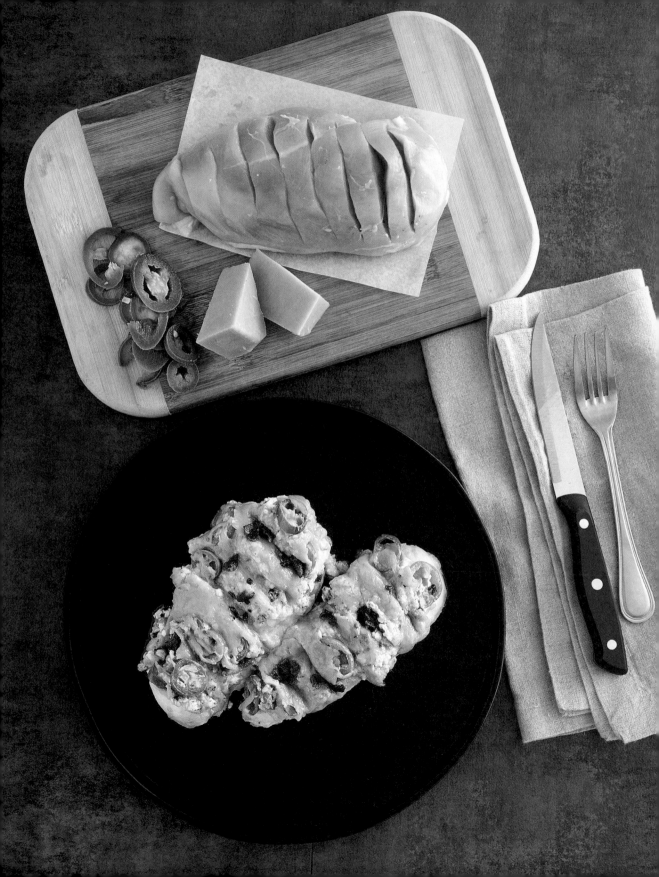

Jalapeño Popper Hasselback Chicken

This easy entrée has plenty of jalapeño spice, but it's complemented by the cream cheese that also keeps the chicken moist and juicy. If you like jalapeño poppers, you'll love this upgraded version!

- **Hands-On Time: 20 minutes**
- **Cook Time: 20 minutes**

Serves 2

4 slices sugar-free bacon, cooked and crumbled

2 ounces full-fat cream cheese, softened

½ cup shredded sharp Cheddar cheese, divided

¼ cup sliced pickled jalapeños

2 (6-ounce) boneless, skinless chicken breasts

TONE DOWN THE SPICE

Not a fan of jalapeños? Try stuffing this chicken with sliced sweet peppers or green bell peppers. You can also make an Italian twist on this dish and stuff with tomato slices and zucchini and sprinkle with Italian seasoning.

1 In a medium bowl, place cooked bacon, then fold in cream cheese, half of the Cheddar, and the jalapeño slices.

2 Use a sharp knife to make slits in each of the chicken breasts about ¾ of the way across the chicken, being careful not to cut all the way through. Depending on the size of the chicken breast, you'll likely have 6–8 slits per breast.

3 Spoon the cream cheese mixture into the slits of the chicken. Sprinkle remaining shredded cheese over chicken breasts and place into the air fryer basket.

4 Adjust the temperature to 350°F and set the timer for 20 minutes.

5 Serve warm.

PER SERVING

CALORIES: 501	**FAT:** 25.3 g
PROTEIN: 53.8 g	**SODIUM:** 860 mg
FIBER: 0.2 g	**CARBOHYDRATES:** 1.6 g
NET CARBOHYDRATES: 1.4 g	**SUGAR:** 1.0 g

Chicken Enchiladas

One great way to make smart swaps in keto recipes is to completely replace an optional high-carb ingredient with a low-carb ingredient that is a major part of the recipe. In this case we're swapping out tortillas for deli chicken so we can still get the full effect without any of the added carbs!

- **Hands-On Time: 20 minutes**
- **Cook Time: 10 minutes**

Serves 4

1½ cups shredded cooked chicken

⅓ cup low-carb enchilada sauce, divided

½ pound medium-sliced deli chicken

1 cup shredded medium Cheddar cheese

½ cup shredded Monterey jack cheese

½ cup full-fat sour cream

1 medium avocado, peeled, pitted, and sliced

1 In a large bowl, mix shredded chicken and half of the enchilada sauce. Lay slices of deli chicken on a work surface and spoon 2 tablespoons shredded chicken mixture onto each slice.

2 Sprinkle 2 tablespoons of Cheddar onto each roll. Gently roll closed.

3 In a 4-cup round baking dish, place each roll, seam side down. Pour remaining sauce over rolls and top with Monterey jack. Place dish into the air fryer basket.

4 Adjust the temperature to 370°F and set the timer for 10 minutes.

5 Enchiladas will be golden on top and bubbling when cooked. Serve warm with sour cream and sliced avocado.

PER SERVING

CALORIES: 416

PROTEIN: 34.2 g

FIBER: 2.3 g

NET CARBOHYDRATES: 4.2 g

FAT: 25.2 g

SODIUM: 1,081 mg

CARBOHYDRATES: 6.5 g

SUGAR: 1.1 g

Chicken Pizza Crust

Using chicken as a pizza crust is a great way to replace carbs with protein! This highly customizable recipe can satisfy your pizza cravings while helping to keep your muscles strong. Even better, it crisps up so well in your air fryer that you can even pick it up just like a traditional slice!

- **Hands-On Time: 10 minutes**
- **Cook Time: 25 minutes**

Serves 4

1 pound ground chicken thigh meat
¼ cup grated Parmesan cheese
½ cup shredded mozzarella

MAKE IT YOUR OWN!
The possibilities for topping this crust are endless! You can add bacon and barbecue sauce for a barbecue chicken pizza or taco seasoning and fresh tomatoes for a Mexican-style pizza. Those are just a couple ideas to get you started!

1 In a large bowl, mix all ingredients. Separate into four even parts.

2 Cut out four (6") circles of parchment and press each portion of the chicken mixture out onto one of the circles. Place into the air fryer basket, working in batches as needed.

3 Adjust the temperature to 375°F and set the timer for 25 minutes.

4 Flip the crust halfway through the cooking time.

5 Once fully cooked, you may top it with cheese and your favorite toppings and cook 5 additional minutes. Or, you may place crust into refrigerator or freezer and top when ready to eat.

PER SERVING

CALORIES: 230	FAT: 12.8 g
PROTEIN: 24.7 g	SODIUM: 268 mg
FIBER: 0.0 g	CARBOHYDRATES: 1.2 g
NET CARBOHYDRATES: 1.2 g	SUGAR: 0.2 g

Blackened Cajun Chicken Tenders

Blackening meat is a technique used to maximize flavor without needing to add any breading. The secret to this chicken is all of the delicious spices that will have you salivating while it cooks!

- **Hands-On Time:** 10 minutes
- **Cook Time:** 17 minutes

Serves 4

2 teaspoons paprika

1 teaspoon chili powder

½ teaspoon garlic powder

½ teaspoon dried thyme

¼ teaspoon onion powder

⅛ teaspoon ground cayenne pepper

2 tablespoons coconut oil

1 pound boneless, skinless chicken tenders

¼ cup full-fat ranch dressing

1 In a small bowl, combine all seasonings.

2 Drizzle oil over chicken tenders and then generously coat each tender in the spice mixture. Place tenders into the air fryer basket.

3 Adjust the temperature to 375°F and set the timer for 17 minutes.

4 Tenders will be 165°F internally when fully cooked. Serve with ranch dressing for dipping.

PER SERVING

CALORIES: 163

PROTEIN: 21.2 g

FIBER: 0.8 g

NET CARBOHYDRATES: 0.7 g

FAT: 7.5 g

SODIUM: 132 mg

CARBOHYDRATES: 1.5 g

SUGAR: 0.2 g

Spinach and Feta–Stuffed Chicken Breast

Stuffing chicken is one of the easiest ways to elevate it. If you need to take your protein to the next level, this recipe is a great creamy and nutritious way to do just that! It comes out deliciously golden brown with hot, gooey, bubbly cheese.

- **Hands-On Time: 15 minutes**
- **Cook Time: 25 minutes**

Serves 2

1 tablespoon unsalted butter

5 ounces frozen spinach, thawed and drained

½ teaspoon garlic powder, divided

½ teaspoon salt, divided

¼ cup chopped yellow onion

¼ cup crumbled feta

2 (6-ounce) boneless, skinless chicken breasts

1 tablespoon coconut oil

1 In a medium skillet over medium heat, add butter to the pan and sauté spinach 3 minutes. Sprinkle ¼ teaspoon garlic powder and ¼ teaspoon salt onto spinach and add onion to the pan.

2 Continue sautéing 3 more minutes, then remove from heat and place in medium bowl. Fold feta into spinach mixture.

3 Slice a roughly 4" slit into the side of each chicken breast, lengthwise. Spoon half of the mixture into each piece and secure closed with a couple toothpicks. Sprinkle outside of chicken with remaining garlic powder and salt. Drizzle with coconut oil. Place chicken breasts into the air fryer basket.

4 Adjust the temperature to 350°F and set the timer for 25 minutes.

5 When completely cooked chicken should be golden brown and have an internal temperature of at least 165°F. Slice and serve warm.

PER SERVING

CALORIES: 393	FAT: 18.5 g
PROTEIN: 43.9 g	SODIUM: 882 mg
FIBER: 2.5 g	CARBOHYDRATES: 6.2 g
NET CARBOHYDRATES: 3.7 g	SUGAR: 2.1 g

Southern "Fried" Chicken

An audible crunch, a juicy middle, and an overflow of flavor are all characteristics of the perfect bite of fried chicken. You'll get all the classic feel you're used to in this favorite without the carbs or the frying oil.

- **Hands-On Time: 15 minutes**
- **Cook Time: 25 minutes**

Serves 4

2 (6-ounce) boneless, skinless chicken breasts
2 tablespoons hot sauce
1 tablespoon chili powder
½ teaspoon cumin
¼ teaspoon onion powder
¼ teaspoon ground black pepper
2 ounces pork rinds, finely ground

1 Slice each chicken breast in half lengthwise. Place the chicken into a large bowl and coat with hot sauce.

2 In a small bowl, mix chili powder, cumin, onion powder, and pepper. Sprinkle over chicken.

3 Place the ground pork rinds into a large bowl and dip each piece of chicken into the bowl, coating as much as possible. Place chicken into the air fryer basket.

4 Adjust the temperature to 350°F and set the timer for 25 minutes.

5 Halfway through the cooking time, carefully flip the chicken.

6 When done, internal temperature will be at least 165°F and pork rind coating will be dark golden brown. Serve warm.

PER SERVING

CALORIES: 192	**FAT:** 6.9 g
PROTEIN: 27.8 g	**SODIUM:** 374 mg
FIBER: 0.9 g	**CARBOHYDRATES:** 1.6 g
NET CARBOHYDRATES: 0.7 g	**SUGAR:** 0.2 g

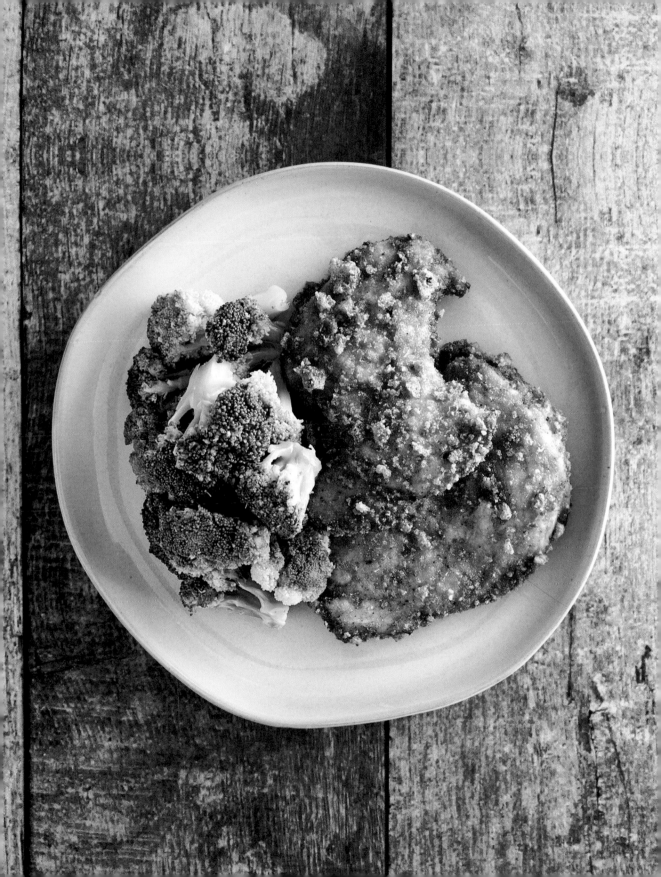

Almond-Crusted Chicken

This chicken comes with a nutty crunch because it's "breaded" with almonds. Not only are almonds a low-carb nut, they are also a fatty, filling food that helps support healthy brain function.

- **Hands-On Time: 15 minutes**
- **Cook Time: 25 minutes**

Serves 4

¼ cup slivered almonds

2 (6-ounce) boneless, skinless chicken breasts

2 tablespoons full-fat mayonnaise

1 tablespoon Dijon mustard

1 Pulse the almonds in a food processor or chop until finely chopped. Place almonds evenly on a plate and set aside.

2 Completely slice each chicken breast in half lengthwise.

3 Mix the mayonnaise and mustard in a small bowl and then coat chicken with the mixture.

4 Lay each piece of chicken in the chopped almonds to fully coat. Carefully move the pieces into the air fryer basket.

5 Adjust the temperature to 350°F and set the timer for 25 minutes.

6 Chicken will be done when it has reached an internal temperature of 165°F or more. Serve warm.

PER SERVING

CALORIES: 195

PROTEIN: 20.9 g

FIBER: 0.8 g

NET CARBOHYDRATES: 1.0 g

FAT: 10.1 g

SODIUM: 175 mg

CARBOHYDRATES: 1.8 g

SUGAR: 0.3 g

Pepperoni and Chicken Pizza Bake

This is a great way to have "pizza" for dinner while piling on the protein! Who could argue with a meal so tasty? This dish will definitely satisfy the whole family while helping to keep everyone's muscles strong!

- **Hands-On Time: 10 minutes**
- **Cook Time: 15 minutes**

Serves 4

2 cups cubed cooked chicken

20 slices pepperoni

1 cup low-carb, sugar-free pizza sauce

1 cup shredded mozzarella cheese

¼ cup grated Parmesan cheese

1 In a 4-cup round baking dish add chicken, pepperoni, and pizza sauce. Stir so meat is completely covered with sauce.

2 Top with mozzarella and grated Parmesan. Place dish into the air fryer basket.

3 Adjust the temperature to 375°F and set the timer for 15 minutes.

4 Dish will be brown and bubbling when cooked. Serve immediately.

PER SERVING

CALORIES: 353	FAT: 17.4 g
PROTEIN: 34.4 g	SODIUM: 754 mg
FIBER: 1.0 g	CARBOHYDRATES: 7.5 g
NET CARBOHYDRATES: 6.5 g	SUGAR: 2.3 g

Quick Chicken Fajitas

Make all the yummy elements of chicken fajitas at the same time with this air fryer spin on a classic sheet pan meal. Serve these with your favorite toppings such as avocado and sour cream. Be sure to pair them with the Pork Rind Tortillas (Chapter 3) for the full effect!

- **Hands-On Time: 10 minutes**
- **Cook Time: 15 minutes**

Serves 2

10 ounces boneless, skinless chicken breast, sliced into ¼" strips

2 tablespoons coconut oil, melted

1 tablespoon chili powder

½ teaspoon cumin

½ teaspoon paprika

½ teaspoon garlic powder

¼ medium onion, peeled and sliced

½ medium green bell pepper, seeded and sliced

½ medium red bell pepper, seeded and sliced

1 Place chicken and coconut oil into a large bowl and sprinkle with chili powder, cumin, paprika, and garlic powder. Toss chicken until well coated with seasoning. Place chicken into the air fryer basket.

2 Adjust the temperature to 350°F and set the timer for 15 minutes.

3 Add onion and peppers into the fryer basket when the timer has 7 minutes remaining.

4 Toss the chicken two or three times during cooking. Vegetables should be tender and chicken fully cooked to at least 165°F internal temperature when finished. Serve warm.

PER SERVING

CALORIES: 326	**FAT:** 15.9 g
PROTEIN: 33.5 g	**SODIUM:** 180 mg
FIBER: 3.2 g	**CARBOHYDRATES:** 8.4 g
NET CARBOHYDRATES: 5.2 g	**SUGAR:** 3.2 g

Chicken Patties

What could be better on a warm summer evening than a juicy burger made from chicken and dredged in crushed pork rinds? This low-carb twist on a classic recipe will leave your whole family satisfied. It's also the perfect meal to prepare ahead of time and freeze for later!

- **Hands-On Time: 15 minutes**
- **Cook Time: 12 minutes**

Serves 4

1 pound ground chicken thigh meat
½ cup shredded mozzarella cheese
1 teaspoon dried parsley
½ teaspoon garlic powder
¼ teaspoon onion powder
1 large egg
2 ounces pork rinds, finely ground

FREEZE IT!

These patties are a great freezer meal for the busy family. Simply "bread" the patties and place them on a parchment-lined baking sheet. Freeze for 2 hours and then place them in a freezer-safe storage bag, separated by parchment squares. Add an additional 5–7 minutes to your cooking time when cooking the frozen patties.

1 In a large bowl, mix ground chicken, mozzarella, parsley, garlic powder, and onion powder. Form into four patties.

2 Place patties in the freezer for 15–20 minutes until they begin to firm up.

3 Whisk egg in a medium bowl. Place the ground pork rinds into a large bowl.

4 Dip each chicken patty into the egg and then press into pork rinds to fully coat. Place patties into the air fryer basket.

5 Adjust the temperature to 360°F and set the timer for 12 minutes.

6 Patties will be firm and cooked to an internal temperature of 165°F when done. Serve immediately.

PER SERVING

CALORIES: 304	**FAT:** 17.4 g
PROTEIN: 32.7 g	**SODIUM:** 406 mg
FIBER: 0.1 g	**CARBOHYDRATES:** 0.9 g
NET CARBOHYDRATES: 0.8 g	**SUGAR:** 0.2 g

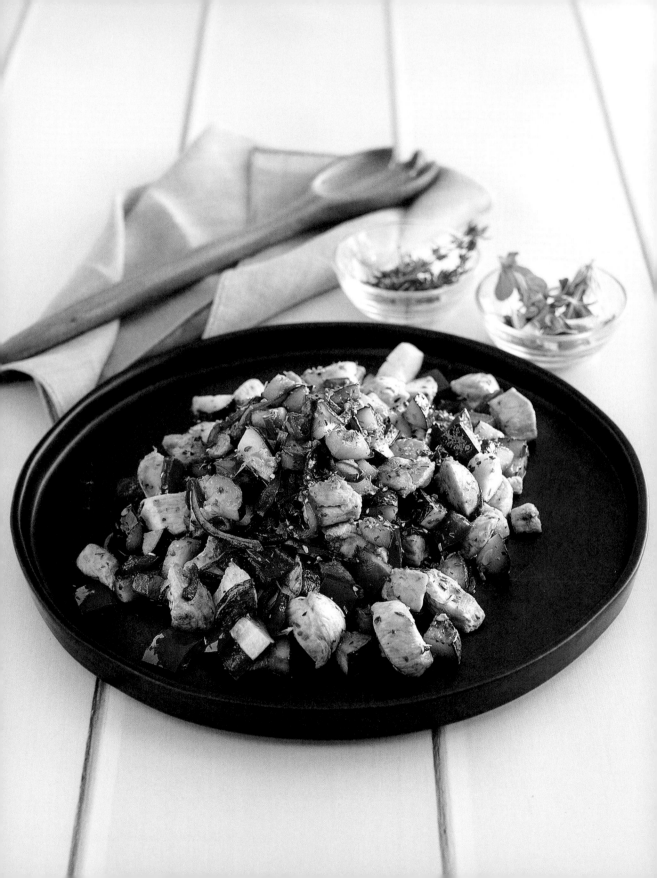

Greek Chicken Stir-Fry

This speedy stir-fry is perfect for a light lunch. For an even more filling meal, try the stir-fry over a bowl of steamed cauliflower!

- **Hands-On Time: 15 minutes**
- **Cook Time: 15 minutes**

Serves 2

1 (6-ounce) chicken breast, cut into 1" cubes
½ medium zucchini, chopped
½ medium red bell pepper, seeded and chopped
¼ medium red onion, peeled and sliced
1 tablespoon coconut oil
1 teaspoon dried oregano
½ teaspoon garlic powder
¼ teaspoon dried thyme

1 Place all ingredients into a large mixing bowl and toss until the coconut oil coats the meat and vegetables. Pour the contents of the bowl into the air fryer basket.

2 Adjust the temperature to 375°F and set the timer for 15 minutes.

3 Shake the fryer basket halfway through the cooking time to redistribute the food. Serve immediately.

PER SERVING

CALORIES: 186	FAT: 8.0 g
PROTEIN: 20.4 g	SODIUM: 43 mg
FIBER: 1.7 g	CARBOHYDRATES: 5.6 g
NET CARBOHYDRATES: 3.9 g	SUGAR: 3.1 g

Chicken, Spinach, and Feta Bites

Combining protein-rich chicken with fiber-filled spinach and calcium-fortified feta cheese makes for a very well-rounded low-carb masterpiece!

- **Hands-On Time: 10 minutes**
- **Cook Time: 12 minutes**

Serves 4

1 pound ground chicken thigh meat
⅓ cup frozen spinach, thawed and drained
⅓ cup crumbled feta
¼ teaspoon onion powder
½ teaspoon garlic powder
½ ounce pork rinds, finely ground

1 Mix all ingredients in a large bowl. Roll into 2" balls and place into the air fryer basket, working in batches if needed.

2 Adjust the temperature to 350°F and set the timer for 12 minutes.

3 When done, internal temperature will be 165°F. Serve immediately.

PER SERVING

CALORIES: 220	FAT: 12.2 g
PROTEIN: 24.1 g	SODIUM: 250 mg
FIBER: 0.4 g	CARBOHYDRATES: 1.5 g
NET CARBOHYDRATES: 1.1 g	SUGAR: 0.6 g

Buffalo Chicken Cheese Sticks

Not only are these cheese sticks ridiculously simple, but they're also very filling. You can thank the added protein from the chicken for turning what is traditionally an appetizer into a satisfying meal.

- **Hands-On Time: 5 minutes**
- **Cook Time: 8 minutes**

Serves 2

1 cup shredded cooked chicken

¼ cup buffalo sauce

1 cup shredded mozzarella cheese

1 large egg

¼ cup crumbled feta

1 In a large bowl, mix all ingredients except the feta. Cut a piece of parchment to fit your air fryer basket and press the mixture into a ½"-thick circle.

2 Sprinkle the mixture with feta and place into the air fryer basket.

3 Adjust the temperature to 400°F and set the timer for 8 minutes.

4 After 5 minutes, flip over the cheese mixture.

5 Allow to cool 5 minutes before cutting into sticks. Serve warm.

PER SERVING

CALORIES: 369

PROTEIN: 35.7 g

FIBER: 0.0 g

NET CARBOHYDRATES: 2.2 g

FAT: 21.5 g

SODIUM: 1,530 mg

CARBOHYDRATES: 2.2 g

SUGAR: 1.4 g

Italian Chicken Thighs

Chicken thighs are ideal for keto cooking. They're generally the most inexpensive part of the chicken and are full of the fat that gives loads of juicy flavor while helping to keep you full. Show off your air fryer's abilities with crispy thighs coated in Italian seasoning!

- **Hands-On Time: 5 minutes**
- **Cook Time: 20 minutes**

Serves 2

4 bone-in, skin-on chicken thighs

2 tablespoons unsalted butter, melted

1 teaspoon dried parsley

1 teaspoon dried basil

½ teaspoon garlic powder

¼ teaspoon onion powder

¼ teaspoon dried oregano

1 Brush chicken thighs with butter and sprinkle remaining ingredients over thighs. Place thighs into the air fryer basket.

2 Adjust the temperature to 380°F and set the timer for 20 minutes.

3 Halfway through the cooking time, flip the thighs.

4 When fully cooked, internal temperature will be at least 165°F and skin will be crispy. Serve warm.

PER SERVING

CALORIES: 596

PROTEIN: 68.3 g

FIBER: 0.4 g

NET CARBOHYDRATES: 0.8 g

FAT: 30.9 g

SODIUM: 292 mg

CARBOHYDRATES: 1.2 g

SUGAR: 0.1 g

Beef and Pork Main Dishes

Beef and pork are two meats, already bursting with flavor, that you can make even better with your air fryer. Who would've thought it would be possible to achieve juicy, tender pork chops in minutes? These versatile meats can be used to create classics in a flash, as well as new and exciting dishes full of healthy protein and fat. With recipes ranging from Bacon Cheeseburger Casserole to Easy Juicy Pork Chops, this chapter will help you beef up your culinary repertoire in no time!

Classic Mini Meatloaf

It seems like meatloaf has been served on dinner tables since the beginning of time. It's a classic dish that many of us remember from childhood. It's also a very easy meal that can be used to hide veggies (for the pickier eaters) without sacrificing a juicy and delicious bite every time.

- **Hands-On Time: 10 minutes**
- **Cook Time: 25 minutes**

Serves 6

1 pound 80/20 ground beef

¼ medium yellow onion, peeled and diced

½ medium green bell pepper, seeded and diced

1 large egg

3 tablespoons blanched finely ground almond flour

1 tablespoon Worcestershire sauce

½ teaspoon garlic powder

1 teaspoon dried parsley

2 tablespoons tomato paste

¼ cup water

1 tablespoon powdered erythritol

1 In a large bowl, combine ground beef, onion, pepper, egg, and almond flour. Pour in the Worcestershire sauce and add the garlic powder and parsley to the bowl. Mix until fully combined.

2 Divide the mixture into two and place into two (4") loaf baking pans.

3 In a small bowl, mix the tomato paste, water, and erythritol. Spoon half the mixture over each loaf.

4 Working in batches if necessary, place loaf pans into the air fryer basket.

5 Adjust the temperature to 350°F and set the timer for 25 minutes or until internal temperature is 180°F.

6 Serve warm.

PER SERVING

CALORIES: 170	**FAT:** 9.4 g
PROTEIN: 14.9 g	**SODIUM:** 85 mg
FIBER: 0.9 g	**CARBOHYDRATES:** 5.0 g
NET CARBOHYDRATES: 2.6 g	**SUGAR:** 1.5 g
SUGAR ALCOHOL: 1.5 g	

Chorizo and Beef Burger

Take burgers to the next level by adding chorizo to the mix! These juicy burgers will be ready to eat in just minutes. If you really miss having them with a bun, you can cut open Dinner Rolls (Chapter 4) and put the burgers inside! Serve these with your favorite burger toppings.

- **Hands-On Time: 10 minutes**
- **Cook Time: 15 minutes**

Serves 4

¾ pound 80/20 ground beef
¼ pound Mexican-style ground chorizo
¼ cup chopped onion
5 slices pickled jalapeños, chopped
2 teaspoons chili powder
1 teaspoon minced garlic
¼ teaspoon cumin

1 In a large bowl, mix all ingredients. Divide the mixture into four sections and form them into burger patties.

2 Place burger patties into the air fryer basket, working in batches if necessary.

3 Adjust the temperature to 375°F and set the timer for 15 minutes.

4 Flip the patties halfway through the cooking time. Serve warm.

PER SERVING

CALORIES: 291	FAT: 18.3 g
PROTEIN: 21.6 g	SODIUM: 474 mg
FIBER: 0.9 g	CARBOHYDRATES: 4.7 g
NET CARBOHYDRATES: 3.8 g	SUGAR: 2.5 g

Crispy Brats

Bratwursts are such a classic summertime lunch, whether you're having a picnic in the backyard or watching a game at the ballpark. And with this recipe you won't even miss the bun! Getting the crunchy, juicy bite that they're known for is easier than ever with your air fryer!

- **Hands-On Time: 5 minutes**
- **Cook Time: 15 minutes**

Serves 4

4 (3-ounce) beef bratwursts

1 Place brats into the air fryer basket.

2 Adjust the temperature to 375°F and set the timer for 15 minutes.

3 Serve warm.

PER SERVING

CALORIES: 286	FAT: 24.8 g
PROTEIN: 11.8 g	SODIUM: 50 mg
FIBER: 0.0 g	CARBOHYDRATES: 0.0 g
NET CARBOHYDRATES: 0.0 g	SUGAR: 0.0 g

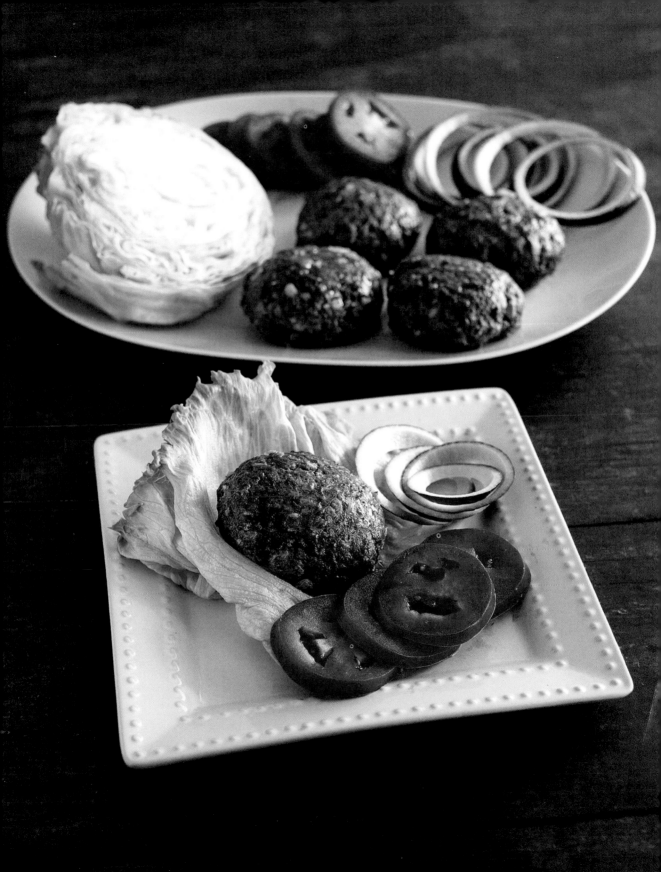

Taco-Stuffed Peppers

You don't have to say goodbye to Taco Tuesday just because you don't eat taco shells anymore. These zesty peppers pack all that classic taco flavor into a pepper instead!

- **Hands-On Time: 15 minutes**
- **Cook Time: 15 minutes**

Serves 4

1 pound 80/20 ground beef

1 tablespoon chili powder

2 teaspoons cumin

1 teaspoon garlic powder

1 teaspoon salt

¼ teaspoon ground black pepper

1 (10-ounce) can diced tomatoes and green chiles, drained

4 medium green bell peppers

1 cup shredded Monterey jack cheese, divided

1 In a medium skillet over medium heat, brown the ground beef about 7–10 minutes. When no pink remains, drain the fat from the skillet.

2 Return the skillet to the stovetop and add chili powder, cumin, garlic powder, salt, and black pepper. Add drained can of diced tomatoes and chiles to the skillet. Continue cooking 3–5 minutes.

3 While the mixture is cooking, cut each bell pepper in half. Remove the seeds and white membrane. Spoon the cooked mixture evenly into each bell pepper and top with a ¼ cup cheese. Place stuffed peppers into the air fryer basket.

4 Adjust the temperature to 350°F and set the timer for 15 minutes.

5 When done, peppers will be fork tender and cheese will be browned and bubbling. Serve warm.

PER SERVING

CALORIES: 346	**FAT:** 19.1 g
PROTEIN: 27.8 g	**SODIUM:** 991 mg
FIBER: 3.5 g	**CARBOHYDRATES:** 10.7 g
NET CARBOHYDRATES: 7.2 g	**SUGAR:** 4.9 g

Italian Stuffed Bell Peppers

Italian seasonings can enhance any dish, and they do just that in these stuffed peppers! With the zesty sausage, the spicy cheese, and the perfect seasonings, this low-carb dish will have your palate pleased!

- **Hands-On Time: 15 minutes**
- **Cook Time: 15 minutes**

Serves 4

1 pound ground pork Italian sausage
½ teaspoon garlic powder
½ teaspoon dried parsley
1 medium Roma tomato, diced
¼ cup chopped onion
4 medium green bell peppers
1 cup shredded mozzarella cheese, divided

1 In a medium skillet over medium heat, brown the ground sausage about 7–10 minutes or until no pink remains. Drain the fat from the skillet.

2 Return the skillet to the stovetop and add garlic powder, parsley, tomato, and onion. Continue cooking 3–5 minutes.

3 Slice peppers in half and remove the seeds and white membrane.

4 Remove the meat mixture from the stovetop and spoon evenly into pepper halves. Top with mozzarella. Place pepper halves into the air fryer basket.

5 Adjust the temperature to 350°F and set the timer for 15 minutes.

6 When done, peppers will be fork tender and cheese will be golden. Serve warm.

PER SERVING

CALORIES: 358	**FAT:** 24.1 g
PROTEIN: 21.1 g	**SODIUM:** 1,029 mg
FIBER: 2.6 g	**CARBOHYDRATES:** 11.3 g
NET CARBOHYDRATES: 8.7 g	**SUGAR:** 4.8 g

Bacon Cheeseburger Casserole

Casseroles are often a favorite for busy people who don't have a lot of time to think about dinner. That's because you can pretty much just put all of the ingredients in a dish and set it to bake. This burger casserole still packs all the flavor of the handheld version. Even better, your air fryer can get this done in a fraction of the time you're used to!

- **Hands-On Time: 15 minutes**
- **Cook Time: 20 minutes**

Serves 4

1 pound 80/20 ground beef

¼ medium white onion, peeled and chopped

1 cup shredded Cheddar cheese, divided

1 large egg

4 slices sugar-free bacon, cooked and crumbled

2 pickle spears, chopped

1 Brown the ground beef in a medium skillet over medium heat about 7–10 minutes. When no pink remains, drain the fat. Remove from heat and add ground beef to large mixing bowl.

2 Add onion, ½ cup Cheddar, and egg to bowl. Mix ingredients well and add crumbled bacon.

3 Pour the mixture into a 4-cup round baking dish and top with remaining Cheddar. Place into the air fryer basket.

4 Adjust the temperature to 375°F and set the timer for 20 minutes.

5 Casserole will be golden on top and firm in the middle when fully cooked. Serve immediately with chopped pickles on top.

PER SERVING

CALORIES: 369

PROTEIN: 31.0 g

FIBER: 0.2 g

NET CARBOHYDRATES: 1.0 g

FAT: 22.6 g

SODIUM: 454 mg

CARBOHYDRATES: 1.2 g

SUGAR: 0.5 g

Pulled Pork

Pulled pork is a barbecue classic. There's nothing better than tender shredded pork slathered in tangy barbecue sauce! Pulled pork is often a slow cooker recipe, with some methods taking more than 8 hours, but if you're short on time, cooking it in your air fryer is the perfect gateway to fast, succulent pork!

- **Hands-On Time: 10 minutes**
- **Cook Time: 2½ hours**

Serves 8

2 tablespoons chili powder
1 teaspoon garlic powder
½ teaspoon onion powder
½ teaspoon ground black pepper
½ teaspoon cumin
1 (4-pound) pork shoulder

1 In a small bowl, mix chili powder, garlic powder, onion powder, pepper, and cumin. Rub the spice mixture over the pork shoulder, patting it into the skin. Place pork shoulder into the air fryer basket.

2 Adjust the temperature to 350°F and set the timer for 150 minutes.

3 Pork skin will be crispy and meat easily shredded with two forks when done. The internal temperature should be at least 145°F.

PER SERVING

CALORIES: 537	**FAT:** 35.5 g
PROTEIN: 42.6 g	**SODIUM:** 180 mg
FIBER: 0.8 g	**CARBOHYDRATES:** 1.5 g
NET CARBOHYDRATES: 0.7 g	**SUGAR:** 0.2 g

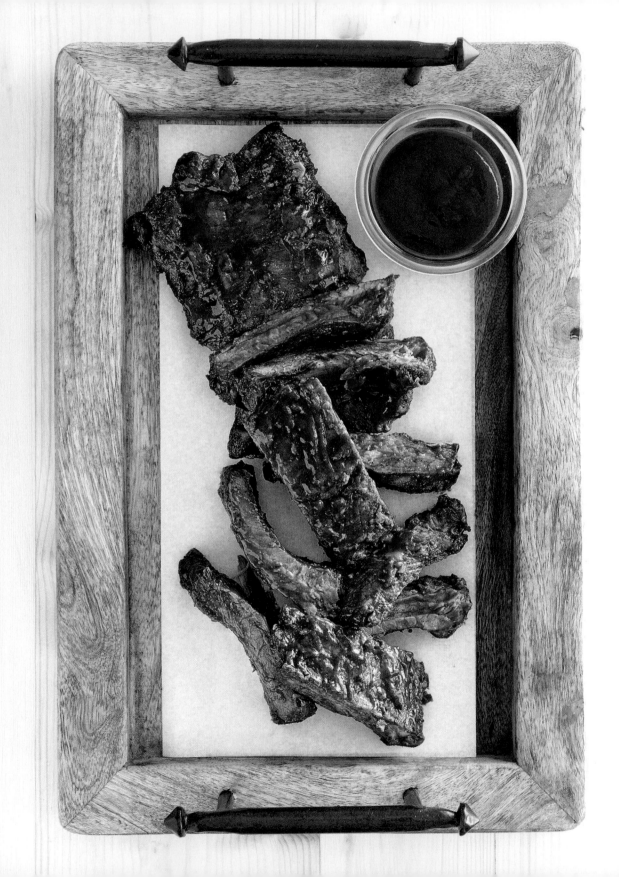

Baby Back Ribs

In a fraction of time, and with none of the bugs from the outdoors, this recipe will make you the grill master of your next barbecue!

- **Hands-On Time: 5 minutes**
- **Cook Time: 25 minutes**

Serves 4

2 pounds baby back ribs
2 teaspoons chili powder
1 teaspoon paprika
½ teaspoon onion powder
½ teaspoon garlic powder
¼ teaspoon ground cayenne pepper
½ cup low-carb, sugar-free barbecue sauce

1 Rub ribs with all ingredients except barbecue sauce. Place into the air fryer basket.

2 Adjust the temperature to 400°F and set the timer for 25 minutes.

3 When done, ribs will be dark and charred with an internal temperature of at least 190°F. Brush ribs with barbecue sauce and serve warm.

PER SERVING

CALORIES: 650	FAT: 51.5 g
PROTEIN: 40.1 g	SODIUM: 332 mg
FIBER: 0.8 g	CARBOHYDRATES: 3.6 g
NET CARBOHYDRATES: 2.8 g	SUGAR: 0.2 g

Bacon-Wrapped Hot Dog

An easy favorite for the family! For a fun twist, try cutting a slit in the top of the hot dog and adding a little cheese before wrapping with the bacon!

- **Hands-On Time: 5 minutes**
- **Cook Time: 10 minutes**

Serves 4

4 beef hot dogs
4 slices sugar-free bacon

1 Wrap each hot dog with slice of bacon and secure with toothpick. Place into the air fryer basket.

2 Adjust the temperature to 370°F and set the timer for 10 minutes.

3 Flip each hot dog halfway through the cooking time. When fully cooked, bacon will be crispy. Serve warm.

PER SERVING

CALORIES: 197	FAT: 15.0 g
PROTEIN: 9.2 g	SODIUM: 571 mg
FIBER: 0.0 g	CARBOHYDRATES: 1.3 g
NET CARBOHYDRATES: 1.3 g	SUGAR: 0.6 g

Easy Juicy Pork Chops

Pork chops are truly one of the easiest main dishes to cook in your air fryer. This cooking technique seals in all the flavorful juices while crisping up the outside for a succulent bite every time. You're just minutes away from pork chop perfection with this recipe!

- **Hands-On Time: 5 minutes**
- **Cook Time: 15 minutes**

Serves 2

1 teaspoon chili powder

½ teaspoon garlic powder

½ teaspoon cumin

¼ teaspoon ground black pepper

¼ teaspoon dried oregano

2 (4-ounce) boneless pork chops

2 tablespoons unsalted butter, divided

1 In a small bowl, mix chili powder, garlic powder, cumin, pepper, and oregano. Rub dry rub onto pork chops. Place pork chops into the air fryer basket.

2 Adjust the temperature to 400°F and set the timer for 15 minutes.

3 The internal temperature should be at least 145°F when fully cooked. Serve warm, each topped with 1 tablespoon butter.

PER SERVING

CALORIES: 313	FAT: 22.6 g
PROTEIN: 24.4 g	SODIUM: 117 mg
FIBER: 0.7 g	CARBOHYDRATES: 1.8 g
NET CARBOHYDRATES: 1.1 g	SUGAR: 0.1 g

SEASONING TIP!

If you're not sure how to season your meat, you can find lots of flavorful dry rubs in your grocery store. Just be sure to check the ingredients carefully as many of these seasonings are loaded with sugar!

Reverse Seared Ribeye

The two main components of a tasty ribeye steak are the juicy inside and the dark sear on the outside. Who would've thought you'd be able to get both in no time with no maintenance at all? This recipe will get you the perfect medium steak, but be sure to adjust the cook time if you prefer yours more or less done!

- **Hands-On Time: 5 minutes**
- **Cook Time: 45 minutes**

Serves 2

1 (8-ounce) ribeye steak
½ teaspoon pink Himalayan salt
¼ teaspoon ground peppercorn
1 tablespoon coconut oil
1 tablespoon salted butter, softened
¼ teaspoon garlic powder
½ teaspoon dried parsley
¼ teaspoon dried oregano

SHORT ON TIME?

You can also quick-cook your ribeye! Place it into the air fryer at 400°F for 10–15 minutes, depending on your preference for doneness. Don't forget to flip halfway through!

1 Rub steak with salt and ground peppercorn. Place into the air fryer basket.

2 Adjust the temperature to 250°F and set the timer for 45 minutes.

3 After timer beeps, begin checking doneness and add a few minutes until internal temperature is your personal preference.

4 In a medium skillet over medium heat, add coconut oil. When oil is hot, quickly sear outside and sides of steak until crisp and browned. Remove from heat and allow steak to rest.

5 In a small bowl, whip butter with garlic powder, parsley, and oregano.

6 Slice steak and serve with herb butter on top.

PER SERVING

CALORIES: 377		**FAT:** 30.7 g
PROTEIN: 22.6 g		**SODIUM:** 490 mg
FIBER: 0.2 g		**CARBOHYDRATES:** 0.6 g
NET CARBOHYDRATES: 0.4 g		**SUGAR:** 0.0 g

Pub-Style Burger

This burger is just bursting with flavor, and it will easily rival any restaurant favorite! After just one bite you'll be ready to kiss those long drive-through lanes goodbye because you'll be able to make your own delicious, much higher-quality burger at home in minutes, thanks to your air fryer!

- **Hands-On Time: 10 minutes**
- **Cook Time: 10 minutes**

Serves 4

1 pound ground sirloin
½ teaspoon salt
¼ teaspoon ground black pepper
2 tablespoons salted butter, melted
½ cup full-fat mayonnaise
2 teaspoons sriracha
¼ teaspoon garlic powder
8 large leaves butter lettuce
4 Bacon-Wrapped Onion Rings (Chapter 3)
8 slices pickle

1 In a medium bowl, combine ground sirloin, salt, and pepper. Form four patties. Brush each with butter and then place into the air fryer basket.

2 Adjust the temperature to 380°F and set the timer for 10 minutes.

3 Flip the patties halfway through the cooking time for a medium burger. Add an additional 3–5 minutes for well-done.

4 In a small bowl, mix mayonnaise, sriracha, and garlic powder. Set aside.

5 Place each cooked burger on a lettuce leaf and top with onion ring, two pickles, and dollop of your prepared burger sauce. Wrap another lettuce leaf around tightly to hold. Serve warm.

PER SERVING

CALORIES: 442	FAT: 34.9 g
PROTEIN: 22.3 g	SODIUM: 928 mg
FIBER: 0.8 g	CARBOHYDRATES: 4.1 g
NET CARBOHYDRATES: 3.3 g	SUGAR: 2.3 g

Pigs in a Blanket

This take on a childhood favorite adds more substance to a plain old hot dog and is the perfect match for your air fryer. Instead of a regular hot dog, which often contains a mixture of poor-quality meats, this recipe uses 100 percent beef sausage, still very low in carbs but a whole lot better for your overall health!

- **Hands-On Time: 10 minutes**
- **Cook Time: 7 minutes**

Serves 2

½ cup shredded mozzarella cheese

2 tablespoons blanched finely ground almond flour

1 ounce full-fat cream cheese

2 (2-ounce) beef smoked sausages

½ teaspoon sesame seeds

CHECK YOUR LABELS!

Some hot dogs can have multiple meats and carb fillers, especially those on the lower price end. Look for hot dogs made from 100 percent beef with 1 carb or less and that have no added fillers, sugar, or gluten. These will usually taste a lot better and are worth the extra couple dollars.

1 Place mozzarella, almond flour, and cream cheese in a large microwave-safe bowl. Microwave for 45 seconds and stir until smooth. Roll dough into a ball and cut in half.

2 Press each half out into a 4" × 5" rectangle. Roll one sausage up in each dough half and press seams closed. Sprinkle the top with sesame seeds.

3 Place each wrapped sausage into the air fryer basket.

4 Adjust the temperature to 400°F and set the timer for 7 minutes.

5 The outside will be golden when completely cooked. Serve immediately.

PER SERVING

CALORIES: 405	**FAT:** 32.2 g
PROTEIN: 17.5 g	**SODIUM:** 693 mg
FIBER: 0.8 g	**CARBOHYDRATES:** 2.9 g
NET CARBOHYDRATES: 2.1 g	**SUGAR:** 1.0 g

Crispy Beef and Broccoli Stir-Fry

You might be surprised to learn that your air fryer is perfect for cooking stir-fry! Temporarily removing your fryer basket and giving it a good shake is a great way to ensure even cooking, or "stir" your dish while it's still cooking.

- **Hands-On Time: 1 hour**
- **Cook Time: 20 minutes**

Serves 2

½ **pound sirloin steak, thinly sliced**

2 **tablespoons soy sauce (or liquid aminos)**

¼ **teaspoon grated ginger**

¼ **teaspoon finely minced garlic**

1 **tablespoon coconut oil**

2 **cups broccoli florets**

¼ **teaspoon crushed red pepper**

⅛ **teaspoon xanthan gum**

½ **teaspoon sesame seeds**

1 To marinate beef, place it into a large bowl or storage bag and add soy sauce, ginger, garlic, and coconut oil. Allow to marinate for 1 hour in refrigerator.

2 Remove beef from marinade, reserving marinade, and place beef into the air fryer basket.

3 Adjust the temperature to 320°F and set the timer for 20 minutes.

4 After 10 minutes, add broccoli and sprinkle red pepper into the fryer basket and shake.

5 Pour the marinade into a skillet over medium heat and bring to a boil, then reduce to simmer. Stir in xanthan gum and allow to thicken.

6 When air fryer timer beeps, quickly empty fryer basket into skillet and toss. Sprinkle with sesame seeds. Serve immediately.

PER SERVING

CALORIES: 342	**FAT:** 18.9 g
PROTEIN: 27.0 g	**SODIUM:** 418 mg
FIBER: 2.7 g	**CARBOHYDRATES:** 9.6 g
NET CARBOHYDRATES: 6.9 g	**SUGAR:** 1.6 g

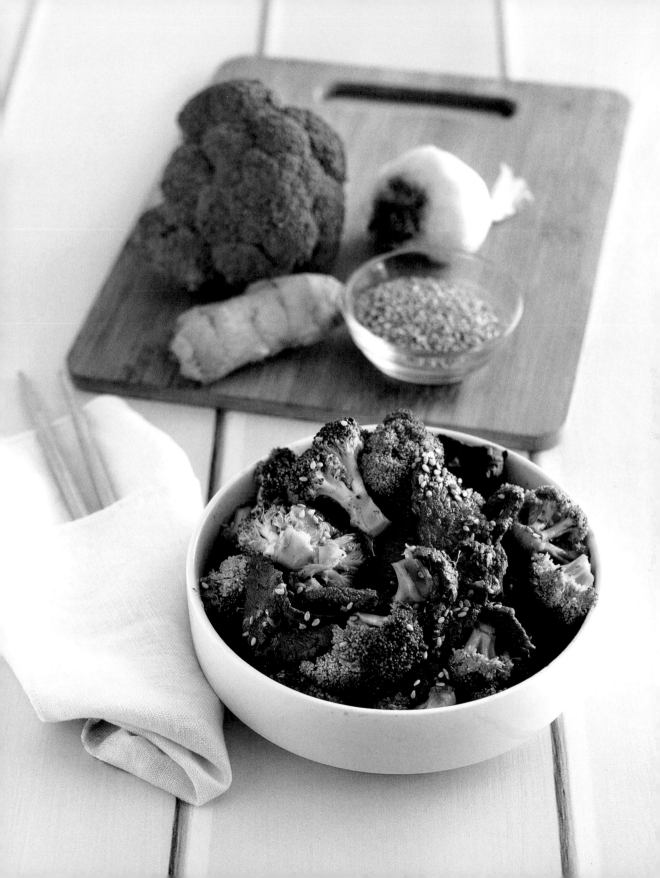

Empanadas

Empanadas are savory Latin American–style pastries usually filled with a Mexican seasoned meat. Serve these with your favorite dipping sauces.

- **Hands-On Time: 15 minutes**
- **Cook Time: 10 minutes**

Yields 4 empanadas (1 per serving)

1 pound 80/20 ground beef
¼ cup water
¼ cup diced onion
2 teaspoons chili powder
½ teaspoon garlic powder
¼ teaspoon cumin
1½ cups shredded mozzarella cheese
½ cup blanched finely ground almond flour
2 ounces full-fat cream cheese
1 large egg

TRICKY DOUGH

Mozzarella dough can be tricky to work with. With practice and patience, you'll find that it can be transformed into everything from pizza crust to crispy coatings to desserts. To handle the dough like an expert, wet your hands with warm water to prevent sticking. Do this as many times as necessary. The excess water will not affect the dough negatively.

1 In a medium skillet over medium heat, brown the ground beef about 7–10 minutes. Drain the fat. Return skillet to stove.

2 Add water and onion to the skillet. Stir and sprinkle with chili powder, garlic powder, and cumin. Reduce heat and simmer an additional 3–5 minutes. Remove from heat and set aside.

3 In a large microwave-safe bowl, add mozzarella, almond flour, and cream cheese. Microwave for 1 minute. Stir until smooth. Form the mixture into a ball.

4 Place dough between two sheets of parchment and roll out to ¼" thickness. Cut the dough into four squares. Place ¼ of ground beef onto the bottom half of each square. Fold the dough over and roll the edges up or press with a wet fork to close.

5 Crack egg into small bowl and whisk. Brush egg over empanadas.

6 Cut a piece of parchment to fit your air fryer basket and place the empanadas on the parchment. Place into the air fryer basket.

7 Adjust the temperature to 400°F and set the timer for 10 minutes.

8 Flip the empanadas halfway through the cooking time. Serve warm.

PER SERVING

CALORIES: 463	**FAT:** 30.8 g
PROTEIN: 33.3 g	**SODIUM:** 426 mg
FIBER: 2.2 g	**CARBOHYDRATES:** 6.5 g
NET CARBOHYDRATES: 4.3 g	**SUGAR:** 1.9 g

Peppercorn-Crusted Beef Tenderloin

This buttery beef tenderloin is deliciously tender and perfectly seasoned with a blend of crushed peppercorns. It's the perfect elevated dish for a special occasion, even though it takes just minutes to prepare!

- **Hands-On Time: 10 minutes**
- **Cook Time: 25 minutes**

Serves 6

2 tablespoons salted butter, melted

2 teaspoons minced roasted garlic

3 tablespoons ground 4-peppercorn blend

1 (2-pound) beef tenderloin, trimmed of visible fat

1 In a small bowl, mix the butter and roasted garlic. Brush it over the beef tenderloin.

2 Place the ground peppercorns onto a plate and roll the tenderloin through them, creating a crust. Place tenderloin into the air fryer basket.

3 Adjust the temperature to 400°F and set the timer for 25 minutes.

4 Turn the tenderloin halfway through the cooking time.

5 Allow meat to rest 10 minutes before slicing.

PER SERVING

CALORIES: 289
PROTEIN: 34.7 g
FIBER: 0.9 g
NET CARBOHYDRATES: 1.6 g

FAT: 13.8 g
SODIUM: 96 mg
CARBOHYDRATES: 2.5 g
SUGAR: 0.0 g

Breaded Pork Chops

Southern-style pork chops aren't complete without a crispy breading. While you wouldn't use flour and bread crumbs on a keto diet, you can definitely make a coating out of more pork...pork rinds! It tastes great and adds zero carbs to your delicious meal!

- **Hands-On Time: 10 minutes**
- **Cook Time: 15 minutes**

Serves 4

1½ ounces pork rinds, finely ground

1 teaspoon chili powder

½ teaspoon garlic powder

1 tablespoon coconut oil, melted

4 (4-ounce) pork chops

1 In a large bowl, mix ground pork rinds, chili powder, and garlic powder.

2 Brush each pork chop with coconut oil and then press into the pork rind mixture, coating both sides. Place each coated pork chop into the air fryer basket.

3 Adjust the temperature to 400°F and set the timer for 15 minutes.

4 Flip each pork chop halfway through the cooking time.

5 When fully cooked the pork chops will be golden on the outside and have an internal temperature of at least 145°F.

PER SERVING

CALORIES: 292	**FAT:** 18.5 g
PROTEIN: 29.5 g	**SODIUM:** 268 mg
FIBER: 0.3 g	**CARBOHYDRATES:** 0.6 g
NET CARBOHYDRATES: 0.3 g	**SUGAR:** 0.1 g

Easy Lasagna Casserole

Forget the layers! This easy casserole is especially for the on-the-go chef who doesn't have time for anything too fancy. You don't miss out on a single lasagna flavor by baking all of the ingredients together, and nobody will know the difference!

- **Hands-On Time: 15 minutes**
- **Cook Time: 15 minutes**

Serves 4

¾ cup low-carb no-sugar-
added pasta sauce

1 pound 80/20 ground beef,
cooked and drained

½ cup full-fat ricotta cheese

¼ cup grated Parmesan
cheese

½ teaspoon garlic powder

1 teaspoon dried parsley

½ teaspoon dried oregano

1 cup shredded mozzarella
cheese

1 In a 4-cup round baking dish, pour ¼ cup pasta sauce on the bottom of the dish. Place ¼ of the ground beef on top of the sauce.

2 In a small bowl, mix ricotta, Parmesan, garlic powder, parsley, and oregano. Place dollops of half the mixture on top of the beef.

3 Sprinkle with ⅓ of the mozzarella. Repeat layers until all beef, ricotta mixture, sauce, and mozzarella are used, ending with the mozzarella on top.

4 Cover dish with foil and place into the air fryer basket.

5 Adjust the temperature to 370°F and set the timer for 15 minutes.

6 In the last 2 minutes of cooking, remove the foil to brown the cheese. Serve immediately.

PER SERVING

CALORIES: 371	**FAT:** 21.4 g
PROTEIN: 31.4 g	**SODIUM:** 633 mg
FIBER: 1.6 g	**CARBOHYDRATES:** 5.8 g
NET CARBOHYDRATES: 4.2 g	**SUGAR:** 1.9 g

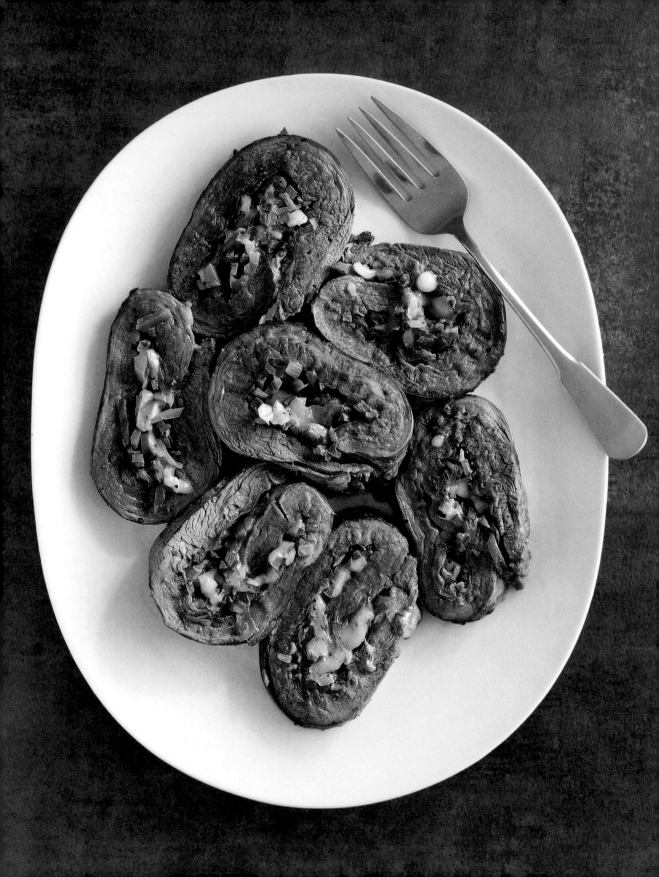

Fajita Flank Steak Rolls

Weekday dinner doesn't have to be boring! These steak rolls come together quickly and can even be prepped the night before. Feel free to switch up the filling with your own favorites, such as spinach with provolone or even Parmesan and asparagus spears.

- **Hands-On Time: 20 minutes**
- **Cook Time: 15 minutes**

Serves 6

2 tablespoons unsalted butter
¼ cup diced yellow onion
1 medium red bell pepper, seeded and sliced into strips
1 medium green bell pepper, seeded and sliced into strips
2 teaspoons chili powder
1 teaspoon cumin
½ teaspoon garlic powder
2 pounds flank steak
4 (1-ounce) slices pepper jack cheese

BUY PREMADE

Short on time? You may be able to find steak rolls freshly made at your grocery store deli! These rolls are becoming more popular, and you might be surprised to find some premade ones at the counter so all you have to do is toss them in the air fryer!

1 In a medium skillet over medium heat, melt butter and begin sautéing onion, red bell pepper, and green bell pepper. Sprinkle with chili powder, cumin, and garlic powder. Sauté until peppers are tender, about 5–7 minutes.

2 Lay flank steak flat on a work surface. Spread onion and pepper mixture over entire steak rectangle. Lay slices of cheese on top of onions and peppers, barely overlapping.

3 With the shortest end toward you, begin rolling the steak, tucking the cheese down into the roll as necessary. Secure the roll with twelve toothpicks, six on each side of the steak roll. Place steak roll into the air fryer basket.

4 Adjust the temperature to 400°F and set the timer for 15 minutes.

5 Rotate the roll halfway through the cooking time. Add an additional 1–4 minutes depending on your preferred internal temperature (135°F for medium).

6 When timer beeps, allow roll to rest 15 minutes, then slice into six even pieces. Serve warm.

PER SERVING

CALORIES: 439	FAT: 26.6 g
PROTEIN: 38.0 g	SODIUM: 226 mg
FIBER: 1.2 g	CARBOHYDRATES: 3.7 g
NET CARBOHYDRATES: 2.5 g	SUGAR: 1.8 g

Ground Beef Taco Rolls

This fun and meaty dish is a Mexican-style spin on an egg roll! Dip these rolls in salsa, sour cream, and guacamole, all low-carb sauces that will enhance the flavor!

- **Hands-On Time: 20 minutes**
- **Cook Time: 10 minutes**

Serves 4

½ pound 80/20 ground beef

⅓ cup water

1 tablespoon chili powder

2 teaspoons cumin

½ teaspoon garlic powder

¼ teaspoon dried oregano

¼ cup canned diced tomatoes and chiles, drained

2 tablespoons chopped cilantro

1½ cups shredded mozzarella cheese

½ cup blanched finely ground almond flour

2 ounces full-fat cream cheese

1 large egg

1 In a medium skillet over medium heat, brown the ground beef about 7–10 minutes. When meat is fully cooked, drain.

2 Add water to skillet and stir in chili powder, cumin, garlic powder, oregano, and tomatoes with chiles. Add cilantro. Bring to a boil, then reduce heat to simmer for 3 minutes.

3 In a large microwave-safe bowl, place mozzarella, almond flour, cream cheese, and egg. Microwave for 1 minute. Stir the mixture quickly until smooth ball of dough forms.

4 Cut a piece of parchment for your work surface. Press the dough into a large rectangle on the parchment, wetting your hands to prevent the dough from sticking as necessary. Cut the dough into eight rectangles.

5 On each rectangle place a few spoons of the meat mixture. Fold the short ends of each roll toward the center and roll the length as you would a burrito.

6 Cut a piece of parchment to fit your air fryer basket. Place taco rolls onto the parchment and place into the air fryer basket.

7 Adjust the temperature to 360°F and set the timer for 10 minutes.

8 Flip halfway through the cooking time.

9 Allow to cool 10 minutes before serving.

PER SERVING

CALORIES: 380	**FAT:** 26.5 g
PROTEIN: 24.8 g	**SODIUM:** 452 mg
FIBER: 2.5 g	**CARBOHYDRATES:** 7.0 g
NET CARBOHYDRATES: 4.5 g	**SUGAR:** 2.0 g

Crispy Pork Chop Salad

It's nearly impossible to overstate the importance of vegetables on a keto diet. They contain key nutrients that help keep your body healthy and functioning properly. One of the best ways to make a salad filling is by adding mouthwatering protein to it. This crispy pork chop salad does just that, and it's something you're going to want to eat every day!

- **Hands-On Time: 15 minutes**
- **Cook Time: 8 minutes**

Serves 2

1 tablespoon coconut oil

2 (4-ounce) pork chops, chopped into 1" cubes

2 teaspoons chili powder

1 teaspoon paprika

½ teaspoon garlic powder

¼ teaspoon onion powder

4 cups chopped romaine

1 medium Roma tomato, diced

½ cup shredded Monterey jack cheese

1 medium avocado, peeled, pitted, and diced

¼ cup full-fat ranch dressing

1 tablespoon chopped cilantro

1 In a large bowl, drizzle coconut oil over pork. Sprinkle with chili powder, paprika, garlic powder, and onion powder. Place pork into the air fryer basket.

2 Adjust the temperature to 400°F and set the timer for 8 minutes.

3 Pork will be golden and crispy when fully cooked.

4 In a large bowl, place romaine, tomato, and crispy pork. Top with shredded cheese and avocado. Pour ranch dressing around bowl and toss the salad to evenly coat.

5 Top with cilantro. Serve immediately.

PER SERVING

CALORIES: 526	FAT: 37.0 g
PROTEIN: 34.4 g	SODIUM: 354 mg
FIBER: 8.6 g	CARBOHYDRATES: 13.8 g
NET CARBOHYDRATES: 5.2 g	SUGAR: 3.1 g

Oversized BBQ Meatballs

These aren't your average meatballs! Supersized, savory, and stuffed with sizzling bacon, they make a filling dinner to satisfy any flavor-loving carnivore!

- **Hands-On Time: 10 minutes**
- **Cook Time: 14 minutes**

Serves 4

1 pound 80/20 ground beef
¼ pound ground Italian
   sausage
1 large egg
¼ teaspoon onion powder
½ teaspoon garlic powder
1 teaspoon dried parsley
4 slices sugar-free bacon,
   cooked and chopped
¼ cup chopped white onion
¼ cup chopped pickled
   jalapeños
½ cup low-carb, sugar-free
   barbecue sauce

1 In a large bowl, mix ground beef, sausage, and egg until fully combined. Mix in all remaining ingredients except barbecue sauce. Form into eight meatballs. Place meatballs into the air fryer basket.

2 Adjust the temperature to 400°F and set the timer for 14 minutes.

3 Turn the meatballs halfway through the cooking time.

4 When done, meatballs should be browned on the outside and have an internal temperature of at least 180°F.

5 Remove meatballs from fryer and toss in barbecue sauce. Serve warm.

PER SERVING

CALORIES: 336
PROTEIN: 28.1 g
FIBER: 0.4 g
NET CARBOHYDRATES: 4.0 g

FAT: 19.5 g
SODIUM: 761 mg
CARBOHYDRATES: 4.4 g
SUGAR: 0.7 g

Fish and Seafood Main Dishes

Get ready to dive into a sea of delicious recipes! Fish is one of the best sources of omega-3 fatty acids, which can help fight inflammation and heart disease, and it's a great source of protein to help keep your muscles strong while you're on a ketogenic diet. Still, despite the flavor and health benefits, seafood is not the easiest cuisine to prepare.

Enter the air fryer. The air fryer will be your favorite tool for creating fresh and delicious, perfectly crisp fish and seafood recipes. From Fried Tuna Salad Bites to Firecracker Shrimp, you'll soon be a master of seafood cuisine, creating flavorful dishes your family can't get enough of!

Lemon Garlic Shrimp

Lemon and garlic are two amazing flavors to complement any seafood. They're simple but create the most mouthwatering blend of sweet, sour, and savory. Pair this shrimp with a bed of zucchini noodles for a more complete meal.

- **Hands-On Time: 5 minutes**
- **Cook Time: 6 minutes**

Serves 2

1 medium lemon

8 ounces medium shelled and deveined shrimp

2 tablespoons unsalted butter, melted

½ teaspoon Old Bay seasoning

½ teaspoon minced garlic

1 Zest lemon and then cut in half. Place shrimp in a large bowl and squeeze juice from ½ lemon on top of them.

2 Add lemon zest to bowl along with remaining ingredients. Toss shrimp until fully coated.

3 Pour bowl contents into 6″ round baking dish. Place into the air fryer basket.

4 Adjust the temperature to 400°F and set the timer for 6 minutes.

5 Shrimp will be bright pink when fully cooked. Serve warm with pan sauce.

PER SERVING

CALORIES: 190	FAT: 11.8 g
PROTEIN: 16.4 g	SODIUM: 812 mg
FIBER: 0.4 g	CARBOHYDRATES: 2.9 g
NET CARBOHYDRATES: 2.5 g	SUGAR: 0.5 g

Cajun Salmon

Salmon can be a bit plain on its own, but that's something you won't have to worry about with this New Orleans–style recipe! The seasonings bring just the right amount of spice to elevate your fish into an irresistible meal!

- **Hands-On Time: 5 minutes**
- **Cook Time: 7 minutes**

Serves 2

2 (4-ounce) salmon fillets, skin removed

2 tablespoons unsalted butter, melted

⅛ teaspoon ground cayenne pepper

½ teaspoon garlic powder

1 teaspoon paprika

¼ teaspoon ground black pepper

1 Brush each fillet with butter.

2 Combine remaining ingredients in a small bowl and then rub onto fish. Place fillets into the air fryer basket.

3 Adjust the temperature to 390°F and set the timer for 7 minutes.

4 When fully cooked, internal temperature will be 145°F. Serve immediately.

PER SERVING

CALORIES: 253	FAT: 16.6 g
PROTEIN: 20.9 g	SODIUM: 46 mg
FIBER: 0.4 g	CARBOHYDRATES: 1.4 g
NET CARBOHYDRATES: 1.0 g	SUGAR: 0.1 g

Blackened Shrimp

This succulent shrimp is just bursting with Cajun flavor. It's a bold and mouthwatering dish that can be eaten on its own or added to a bowl of zucchini noodles for a pasta feel.

- **Hands-On Time: 5 minutes**
- **Cook Time: 6 minutes**

Serves 2

8 ounces medium shelled and deveined shrimp

2 tablespoons salted butter, melted

1 teaspoon paprika

½ teaspoon garlic powder

¼ teaspoon onion powder

½ teaspoon Old Bay seasoning

1 Toss all ingredients together in a large bowl. Place shrimp into the air fryer basket.

2 Adjust the temperature to 400°F and set the timer for 6 minutes.

3 Turn the shrimp halfway through the cooking time to ensure even cooking. Serve immediately.

PER SERVING

CALORIES: 192	FAT: 11.9 g
PROTEIN: 16.6 g	SODIUM: 902 mg
FIBER: 0.5 g	CARBOHYDRATES: 2.5 g
NET CARBOHYDRATES: 2.0 g	SUGAR: 0.2 g

Coconut Shrimp

The coconut in this recipe gives the juicy shrimp a sweet, crispy, golden crust. It's the perfect finger food (paired with sriracha) for a summertime barbecue, or it can also be served on a bed of greens for an easy salad.

- **Hands-On Time: 5 minutes**
- **Cook Time: 6 minutes**

Serves 2

8 ounces medium shelled and deveined shrimp

2 tablespoons salted butter, melted

½ teaspoon Old Bay seasoning

¼ cup unsweetened shredded coconut

THE UNSWEETENED DIFFERENCE

Be sure to buy unsweetened shredded coconut! Sweetened versions are also available, but this recipe avoids unnecessary sugars by relying on the coconut's natural sweetness.

1 In a large bowl, toss the shrimp in butter and Old Bay seasoning.

2 Place shredded coconut in bowl. Coat each piece of shrimp in the coconut and place into the air fryer basket.

3 Adjust the temperature to 400°F and set the timer for 6 minutes.

4 Gently turn the shrimp halfway through the cooking time. Serve immediately.

PER SERVING

CALORIES: 252	FAT: 17.8 g
PROTEIN: 16.9 g	SODIUM: 902 mg
FIBER: 2.0 g	CARBOHYDRATES: 3.8 g
NET CARBOHYDRATES: 1.8 g	SUGAR: 0.7 g

Foil-Packet Salmon

Baking salmon in a foil packet is a great way to steam the meat while locking in the flavors of whichever spices and vegetables you want to cook with it. Typically, this could take up to 30 minutes, but in your air fryer, you'll have perfectly tender salmon in no time!

- **Hands-On Time: 10 minutes**
- **Cook Time: 12 minutes**

Serves 2

2 (4-ounce) salmon fillets, skin removed
2 tablespoons unsalted butter, melted
½ teaspoon garlic powder
1 medium lemon
½ teaspoon dried dill

FOIL MAKES IT EASY!
Foil packets are an easy, no-mess way to cook a meal. You can even eat it right out of the pack! You can put your own twist by swapping out the lemon for lime and adding chili powder or your own favorite seasoning.

1 Place each fillet on a 5" × 5" square of aluminum foil. Drizzle with butter and sprinkle with garlic powder.

2 Zest half of the lemon and sprinkle zest over salmon. Slice other half of the lemon and lay two slices on each piece of salmon. Sprinkle dill over salmon.

3 Gather and fold foil at the top and sides to fully close packets. Place foil packets into the air fryer basket.

4 Adjust the temperature to 400°F and set the timer for 12 minutes.

5 Salmon will be easily flaked and have an internal temperature of at least 145°F when fully cooked. Serve immediately.

PER SERVING

CALORIES: 252	**FAT:** 16.5 g
PROTEIN: 20.9 g	**SODIUM:** 47 mg
FIBER: 0.4 g	**CARBOHYDRATES:** 1.2 g
NET CARBOHYDRATES: 0.8 g	**SUGAR:** 0.2 g

Crispy Fish Sticks

Say goodbye to store-bought! These fish sticks are easy to make, and even freeze well, and they contain none of the high-carb junk (like wheat flour and cornstarch) you'll find in traditional fish sticks. This is a smart swap you'll be proud to feed to your family!

- **Hands-On Time: 15 minutes**
- **Cook Time: 10 minutes**

Serves 4 (4 sticks per serving)

1 ounce pork rinds, finely ground

¼ cup blanched finely ground almond flour

½ teaspoon Old Bay seasoning

1 tablespoon coconut oil

1 large egg

1 pound cod fillet, cut into ¾" strips

FREEZE AHEAD!

This family favorite is a great make-ahead freezer meal! After you coat the fish sticks, place them on a parchment-lined baking sheet, leaving space in between, and freeze them for 2 hours. Once frozen, place them in an airtight sealed storage bag. Just add 4–5 minutes to the cook time if making from frozen sticks.

1 Place ground pork rinds, almond flour, Old Bay seasoning, and coconut oil into a large bowl and mix together. In a medium bowl, whisk egg.

2 Dip each fish stick into the egg and then gently press into the flour mixture, coating as fully and evenly as possible. Place fish sticks into the air fryer basket.

3 Adjust the temperature to 400°F and set the timer for 10 minutes or until golden.

4 Serve immediately.

PER SERVING

CALORIES: 205	FAT: 10.7 g
PROTEIN: 24.4 g	SODIUM: 547 mg
FIBER: 0.8 g	CARBOHYDRATES: 1.6 g
NET CARBOHYDRATES: 0.8 g	SUGAR: 0.3 g

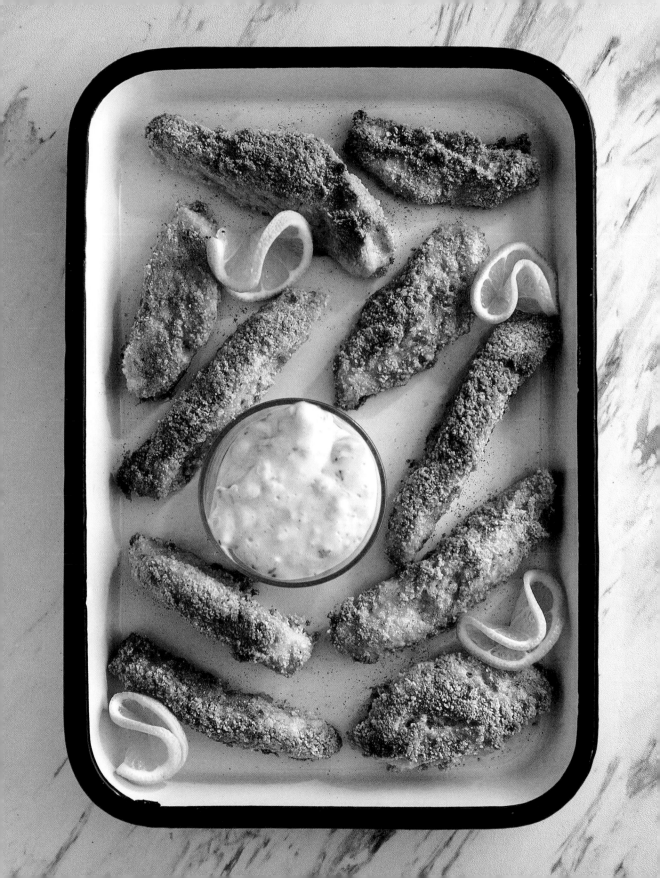

Salmon Patties

Salmon Patties, or salmon cakes, are like a fish burger full of heart-healthy omega-3 fatty acids. They're a delicious meal that is best served in a lettuce wrap. You'll want to opt for a wild-caught salmon because this variety helps you to avoid many of the contaminants that farmed salmon often carry.

- **Hands-On Time: 10 minutes**
- **Cook Time: 8 minutes**

Serves 2

2 (5-ounce) pouches cooked pink salmon

1 large egg

¼ cup ground pork rinds

2 tablespoons full-fat mayonnaise

2 teaspoons sriracha

1 teaspoon chili powder

1 Mix all ingredients in a large bowl and form into four patties. Place patties into the air fryer basket.

2 Adjust the temperature to 400°F and set the timer for 8 minutes.

3 Carefully flip each patty halfway through the cooking time. Patties will be crispy on the outside when fully cooked.

PER SERVING

CALORIES: 319	FAT: 19.0 g
PROTEIN: 33.8 g	SODIUM: 843 mg
FIBER: 0.5 g	CARBOHYDRATES: 1.9 g
NET CARBOHYDRATES: 1.4 g	SUGAR: 1.3 g

THE PERFECT BINDER

Instead of bread crumbs, which are high in carbs, you can make a binder using ground pork rinds. Simply empty the bag into your food processor and pulse until it's a flour or dust consistency. This will hold your meats together just as well as a wheat flour without any added carbs!

Firecracker Shrimp

This dish packs some serious heat! It's perfect for lovers of seafood who can't get enough spice in their life. The secret behind the flavor is hot chili sauce, also known as sriracha. It can be found in any grocery store and has only 1 gram of carbs per serving!

- **Hands-On Time: 10 minutes**
- **Cook Time: 7 minutes**

Serves 4

1 pound medium shelled and deveined shrimp

2 tablespoons salted butter, melted

½ teaspoon Old Bay seasoning

¼ teaspoon garlic powder

2 tablespoons sriracha

¼ teaspoon powdered erythritol

¼ cup full-fat mayonnaise

⅛ teaspoon ground black pepper

1 In a large bowl, toss shrimp in butter, Old Bay seasoning, and garlic powder. Place shrimp into the air fryer basket.

2 Adjust the temperature to 400°F and set the timer for 7 minutes.

3 Flip the shrimp halfway through the cooking time. Shrimp will be bright pink when fully cooked.

4 In another large bowl, mix sriracha, powdered erythritol, mayonnaise, and pepper. Toss shrimp in the spicy mixture and serve immediately.

PER SERVING

CALORIES: 143	**FAT:** 6.4 g
PROTEIN: 16.4 g	**SODIUM:** 936 mg
FIBER: 0.0 g	**CARBOHYDRATES:** 3.0 g
NET CARBOHYDRATES: 2.8 g	**SUGAR:** 1.5 g
SUGAR ALCOHOL: 0.2 g	

Crab Legs

Grab your garlic butter! It'll be perfect for dipping your succulent Crab Legs. This crustaceous creation bakes up beautifully in your air fryer, and you can even use the crabmeat to make the Hot Crab Dip (see recipe in this chapter)!

- **Hands-On Time: 5 minutes**
- **Cook Time: 15 minutes**

Serves 4

¼ cup salted butter, melted and divided

3 pounds crab legs

¼ teaspoon garlic powder

Juice of ½ medium lemon

1. In a large bowl, drizzle 2 tablespoons butter over crab legs. Place crab legs into the air fryer basket.

2. Adjust the temperature to 400°F and set the timer for 15 minutes.

3. Shake the air fryer basket to toss the crab legs halfway through the cooking time.

4. In a small bowl, mix remaining butter, garlic powder, and lemon juice.

5. To serve, crack open crab legs and remove meat. Dip in lemon butter.

PER SERVING

CALORIES: 123	**FAT:** 5.6 g
PROTEIN: 15.7 g	**SODIUM:** 756 mg
FIBER: 0.0 g	**CARBOHYDRATES:** 0.4 g
NET CARBOHYDRATES: 0.4 g	**SUGAR:** 0.1 g

Foil-Packet Lobster Tail

Convince anyone you're a master chef or perfectly set the mood for a romantic dinner with this beautifully steamed lobster tail! From a health standpoint, lobster is also rich in vitamin B, which plays a vital role in your body's metabolism.

- **Hands-On Time: 15 minutes**
- **Cook Time: 12 minutes**

Serves 2

2 (6-ounce) lobster tails, halved

2 tablespoons salted butter, melted

½ teaspoon Old Bay seasoning

Juice of ½ medium lemon

1 teaspoon dried parsley

1 Place the two halved tails on a sheet of aluminum foil. Drizzle with butter, Old Bay seasoning, and lemon juice.

2 Seal the foil packets, completely covering tails. Place into the air fryer basket.

3 Adjust the temperature to 375°F and set the timer for 12 minutes.

4 Once done, sprinkle with dried parsley and serve immediately.

PER SERVING

CALORIES: 234	**FAT:** 11.9 g
PROTEIN: 28.3 g	**SODIUM:** 951 mg
FIBER: 0.1 g	**CARBOHYDRATES:** 0.7 g
NET CARBOHYDRATES: 0.6 g	**SUGAR:** 0.2 g

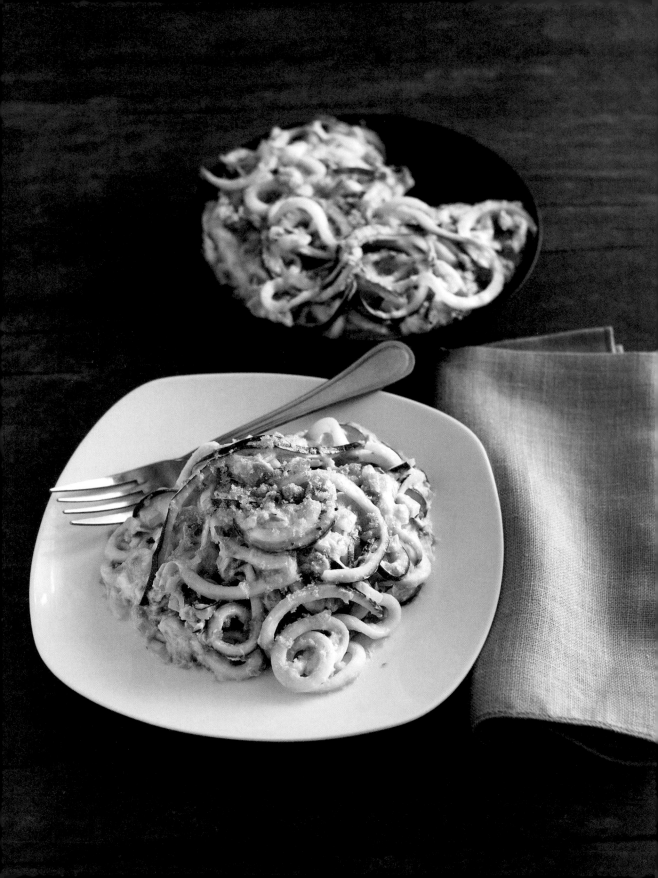

Tuna Zoodle Casserole

This is a dish the whole family will love! The spiralized zucchini tossed in three different types of cheese makes this a gooey, delicious, and filling meal. You'll want to choose a spiralizer model based on how frequently you think you'll use it. Handheld spiralizers are great for small portions, but if you make large bowls for the family, then counter-mounted spiralizers with a crank are an excellent option.

- **Hands-On Time: 15 minutes**
- **Cook Time: 15 minutes**

Serves 4

2 tablespoons salted butter

¼ cup diced white onion

¼ cup chopped white mushrooms

2 stalks celery, finely chopped

½ cup heavy cream

½ cup vegetable broth

2 tablespoons full-fat mayonnaise

¼ teaspoon xanthan gum

½ teaspoon red pepper flakes

2 medium zucchini, spiralized

2 (5-ounce) cans albacore tuna

1 ounce pork rinds, finely ground

1 In a large saucepan over medium heat, melt butter. Add onion, mushrooms, and celery and sauté until fragrant, about 3–5 minutes.

2 Pour in heavy cream, vegetable broth, mayonnaise, and xanthan gum. Reduce heat and continue cooking an additional 3 minutes, until the mixture begins to thicken.

3 Add red pepper flakes, zucchini, and tuna. Turn off heat and stir until zucchini noodles are coated.

4 Pour into 4-cup round baking dish. Top with ground pork rinds and cover the top of the dish with foil. Place into the air fryer basket.

5 Adjust the temperature to 370°F and set the timer for 15 minutes.

6 When 3 minutes remain, remove the foil to brown the top of the casserole. Serve warm.

PER SERVING

CALORIES: 339

PROTEIN: 19.7 g

FIBER: 1.8 g

NET CARBOHYDRATES: 4.3 g

FAT: 25.1 g

SODIUM: 522 mg

CARBOHYDRATES: 6.1 g

SUGAR: 4.1 g

Shrimp Scampi

You won't believe how quickly this succulent and tender Shrimp Scampi comes together. None of the buttery goodness dries out in your air fryer, so you can serve it in the sauce it cooks in!

- **Hands-On Time:** 10 minutes
- **Cook Time:** 8 minutes

Serves 4

4 tablespoons salted butter

½ medium lemon

1 teaspoon minced roasted garlic

¼ cup heavy whipping cream

¼ teaspoon xanthan gum

¼ teaspoon red pepper flakes

1 pound medium peeled and deveined shrimp

1 tablespoon chopped fresh parsley

1 In a medium saucepan over medium heat, melt butter. Zest the lemon, then squeeze juice into the pan. Add garlic.

2 Pour in the cream, xanthan gum, and red pepper flakes. Whisk until the mixture begins to thicken, about 2–3 minutes.

3 Place shrimp into a 4-cup round baking dish. Pour the cream sauce over the shrimp and cover with foil. Place the dish into the air fryer basket.

4 Adjust the temperature to 400°F and set the timer for 8 minutes.

5 Stir twice during cooking.

6 When done, garnish with parsley and serve warm.

PER SERVING

CALORIES: 240

PROTEIN: 16.7 g

FIBER: 0.4 g

NET CARBOHYDRATES: 2.0 g

FAT: 17.0 g

SODIUM: 769 mg

CARBOHYDRATES: 2.4 g

SUGAR: 0.6 g

Fried Tuna Salad Bites

This is a recipe even the little ones will love! It's a great alternative to fish sticks and is full of nutrients and fiber from the avocado. These bites have all the flavors of a traditional tuna salad with a crunchy outside that will keep the kids coming back for more.

- **Hands-On Time: 10 minutes**
- **Cook Time: 7 minutes**

**Yields 12 bites
(3 per serving)**

1 (10-ounce) can tuna, drained

¼ cup full-fat mayonnaise

1 stalk celery, chopped

1 medium avocado, peeled, pitted, and mashed

½ cup blanched finely ground almond flour, divided

2 teaspoons coconut oil

SPICE IT UP!

Add some spice to this dish by adding 2 teaspoons of sriracha to the mayonnaise. Sriracha is a sauce made from chiles, vinegar, sugar, and salt. Even though it does have some sugar, it's generally fine to eat because a small amount goes a long way in a recipe. Some brands have more added sugar than others, so look for one with the smallest amount.

1 In a large bowl, mix tuna, mayonnaise, celery, and mashed avocado. Form the mixture into balls.

2 Roll balls in almond flour and spritz with coconut oil. Place balls into the air fryer basket.

3 Adjust the temperature to 400°F and set the timer for 7 minutes.

4 Gently turn tuna bites after 5 minutes. Serve warm.

PER SERVING

CALORIES: 323		FAT: 25.4 g	
PROTEIN: 17.3 g		SODIUM: 311 mg	
FIBER: 4.0 g		CARBOHYDRATES: 6.3 g	
NET CARBOHYDRATES: 2.3 g		SUGAR: 0.8 g	

Fish Taco Bowl with Jalapeño Slaw

This spicy taco bowl is a great change from beef or chicken. If you've been missing that taco crunch, the slaw will satisfy your craving. The crunchy cabbage paired with a creamy sauce and tart lime make this a memorable dish. If spicy isn't your thing, feel free to omit the jalapeños and add your favorite toppings!

- **Hands-On Time: 10 minutes**
- **Cook Time: 10 minutes**

Serves 2

1 cup shredded cabbage
¼ cup full-fat sour cream
2 tablespoons full-fat mayonnaise
¼ cup chopped pickled jalapeños
2 (3-ounce) cod fillets
1 teaspoon chili powder
1 teaspoon cumin
½ teaspoon paprika
¼ teaspoon garlic powder
1 medium avocado, peeled, pitted, and sliced
½ medium lime

1 In a large bowl, place cabbage, sour cream, mayonnaise, and jalapeños. Mix until fully coated. Let sit for 20 minutes in the refrigerator.

2 Sprinkle cod fillets with chili powder, cumin, paprika, and garlic powder. Place each fillet into the air fryer basket.

3 Adjust the temperature to 370°F and set the timer for 10 minutes.

4 Flip the fillets halfway through the cooking time. When fully cooked, fish should have an internal temperature of at least 145°F.

5 To serve, divide slaw mixture into two serving bowls, break cod fillets into pieces and spread over the bowls, and top with avocado. Squeeze lime juice over each bowl. Serve immediately.

PER SERVING

CALORIES: 342	FAT: 25.2 g
PROTEIN: 16.1 g	SODIUM: 587 mg
FIBER: 6.4 g	CARBOHYDRATES: 11.7 g
NET CARBOHYDRATES: 5.3 g	SUGAR: 2.8 g

Hot Crab Dip

This creamy dip comes together very quickly and is a crowd-pleaser! The hot sauce and jalapeños add a nice kick to this otherwise creamy dip. Serve with sliced cucumbers or pork rinds for dipping.

- **Hands-On Time: 10 minutes**
- **Cook Time: 8 minutes**

Serves 4

8 ounces full-fat cream cheese, softened

¼ cup full-fat mayonnaise

¼ cup full-fat sour cream

1 tablespoon lemon juice

½ teaspoon hot sauce

¼ cup chopped pickled jalapeños

¼ cup sliced green onion

2 (6-ounce) cans lump crabmeat

½ cup shredded Cheddar cheese

1 Place all ingredients into a 4-cup round baking dish and stir until fully combined. Place dish into the air fryer basket.

2 Adjust the temperature to 400°F and set the timer for 8 minutes.

3 Dip will be bubbling and hot when done. Serve warm.

PER SERVING

CALORIES: 441	FAT: 33.8 g
PROTEIN: 17.8 g	SODIUM: 791 mg
FIBER: 0.6 g	CARBOHYDRATES: 8.2 g
NET CARBOHYDRATES: 7.6 g	SUGAR: 6.6 g

Almond Pesto Salmon

Both almonds and salmon are great sources of healthy fat. The almonds add a nice crunch to this dish, and the pesto brings out the natural flavors of the salmon. While basil might not immediately come to your mind when you think of fish, it adds a nice freshness to this warm dish.

- **Hands-On Time: 5 minutes**
- **Cook Time: 12 minutes**

Serves 2

¼ cup pesto

¼ cup sliced almonds, roughly chopped

2 (1½"-thick) salmon fillets (about 4 ounces each)

2 tablespoons unsalted butter, melted

1 In a small bowl, mix pesto and almonds. Set aside.

2 Place fillets into a 6″ round baking dish.

3 Brush each fillet with butter and place half of the pesto mixture on the top of each fillet. Place dish into the air fryer basket.

4 Adjust the temperature to 390°F and set the timer for 12 minutes.

5 Salmon will easily flake when fully cooked and reach an internal temperature of at least 145°F. Serve warm.

PER SERVING

CALORIES: 433	**FAT:** 34.0 g
PROTEIN: 23.3 g	**SODIUM:** 341 mg
FIBER: 2.4 g	**CARBOHYDRATES:** 6.1 g
NET CARBOHYDRATES: 3.7 g	**SUGAR:** 0.9 g

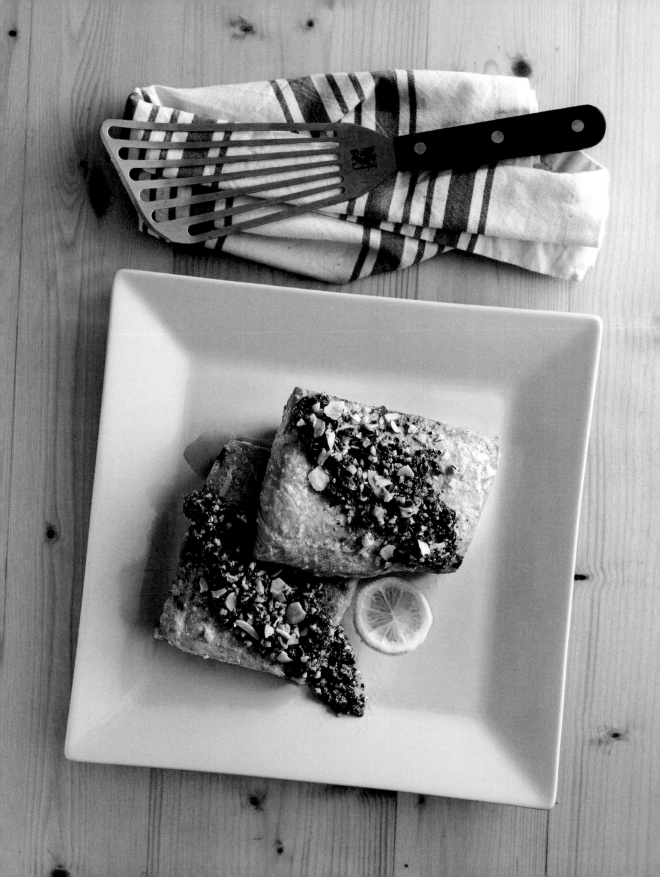

Crab Cakes

These cakes have all the flavor of a traditional crab cake with much fewer carbs. Usually bread crumbs or wheat flour is added as a binder, but this version cuts the carbs by using almond flour. It doesn't change the taste and will make the cakes much easier to flip than completely leaving out a binder would.

- **Hands-On Time: 10 minutes**
- **Cook Time: 10 minutes**

Serves 4

2 (6-ounce) cans lump crabmeat

¼ cup blanched finely ground almond flour

1 large egg

2 tablespoons full-fat mayonnaise

½ teaspoon Dijon mustard

½ tablespoon lemon juice

½ medium green bell pepper, seeded and chopped

¼ cup chopped green onion

½ teaspoon Old Bay seasoning

1 In a large bowl, combine all ingredients. Form into four balls and flatten into patties. Place patties into the air fryer basket.

2 Adjust the temperature to 350°F and set the timer for 10 minutes.

3 Flip patties halfway through the cooking time. Serve warm.

PER SERVING

CALORIES: 151	FAT: 10.0 g
PROTEIN: 13.4 g	SODIUM: 467 mg
FIBER: 0.9 g	CARBOHYDRATES: 2.3 g
NET CARBOHYDRATES: 1.4 g	SUGAR: 0.5 g

MAKE IT FRESH!

Fresh crabmeat can also be used for these cakes. Check out the Crab Legs recipe in this chapter to learn how to make quick and easy crab legs in your air fryer!

Cilantro Lime Baked Salmon

Whether you haven't cooked fish before or have been cooking it for years, this is a great staple recipe. The cilantro adds a freshness that is complemented well by the tartness of the lime. Try this dish with riced cauliflower or steamed veggies and everyone will be asking for seconds.

- **Hands-On Time: 10 minutes**
- **Cook Time: 12 minutes**

Serves 2

2 (3-ounce) salmon fillets, skin removed

1 tablespoon salted butter, melted

1 teaspoon chili powder

½ teaspoon finely minced garlic

¼ cup sliced pickled jalapeños

½ medium lime, juiced

2 tablespoons chopped cilantro

1 Place salmon fillets into a 6" round baking pan. Brush each with butter and sprinkle with chili powder and garlic.

2 Place jalapeño slices on top and around salmon. Pour half of the lime juice over the salmon and cover with foil. Place pan into the air fryer basket.

3 Adjust the temperature to 370°F and set the timer for 12 minutes.

4 When fully cooked, salmon should flake easily with a fork and reach an internal temperature of at least 145°F.

5 To serve, spritz with remaining lime juice and garnish with cilantro.

PER SERVING

CALORIES: 167	FAT: 9.9 g
PROTEIN: 15.8 g	SODIUM: 248 mg
FIBER: 0.7 g	CARBOHYDRATES: 1.6 g
NET CARBOHYDRATES: 0.9 g	SUGAR: 0.2 g

Sesame-Crusted Tuna Steak

Tuna is a very mild-tasting fish, which is great for those new to seafood. This dish is very simple to prepare and gives you a much deeper flavor than canned tuna. While some prefer their tuna steaks well-done and flaky, others enjoy a medium-rare tuna steak, which is still safe to eat. Make sure you buy your tuna steak fresh and avoid leaving it uncooked for more than a couple days in the refrigerator.

- **Hands-On Time: 5 minutes**
- **Cook Time: 8 minutes**

Serves 2

2 (6-ounce) tuna steaks

1 tablespoon coconut oil, melted

½ teaspoon garlic powder

2 teaspoons white sesame seeds

2 teaspoons black sesame seeds

1 Brush each tuna steak with coconut oil and sprinkle with garlic powder.

2 In a large bowl, mix sesame seeds and then press each tuna steak into them, covering the steak as completely as possible. Place tuna steaks into the air fryer basket.

3 Adjust the temperature to 400°F and set the timer for 8 minutes.

4 Flip the steaks halfway through the cooking time. Steaks will be well-done at 145°F internal temperature. Serve warm.

PER SERVING

CALORIES: 280	**FAT:** 10.0 g
PROTEIN: 42.7 g	**SODIUM:** 77 mg
FIBER: 0.8 g	**CARBOHYDRATES:** 2.0 g
NET CARBOHYDRATES: 1.2 g	**SUGAR:** 0.0 g

Spicy Salmon Jerky

Jerky isn't just for beef anymore! Salmon jerky is gaining popularity and rightfully so because it's full of so many great nutrients. It's good on the go but can also be used chopped up as a salad topper or served as an appetizer alongside whipped cream cheese.

- **Hands-On Time: 5 minutes**
- **Cook Time: 4 hours**

Serves 4

1 pound salmon, skin and bones removed
¼ cup soy sauce (or liquid aminos)
½ teaspoon liquid smoke
¼ teaspoon ground black pepper
Juice of ½ medium lime
½ teaspoon ground ginger
¼ teaspoon red pepper flakes

1 Slice salmon into ¼"-thick slices, 4" long.

2 Place strips into a large storage bag or a covered bowl and add remaining ingredients. Allow to marinate for 2 hours in the refrigerator.

3 Place each strip into the air fryer basket in a single layer.

4 Adjust the temperature to 140°F and set the timer for 4 hours.

5 Cool then store in a sealed container until ready to eat.

PER SERVING

CALORIES: 108	**FAT:** 4.1 g
PROTEIN: 15.1 g	**SODIUM:** 469 mg
FIBER: 0.2 g	**CARBOHYDRATES:** 1.0 g
NET CARBOHYDRATES: 0.8 g	**SUGAR:** 0.1 g

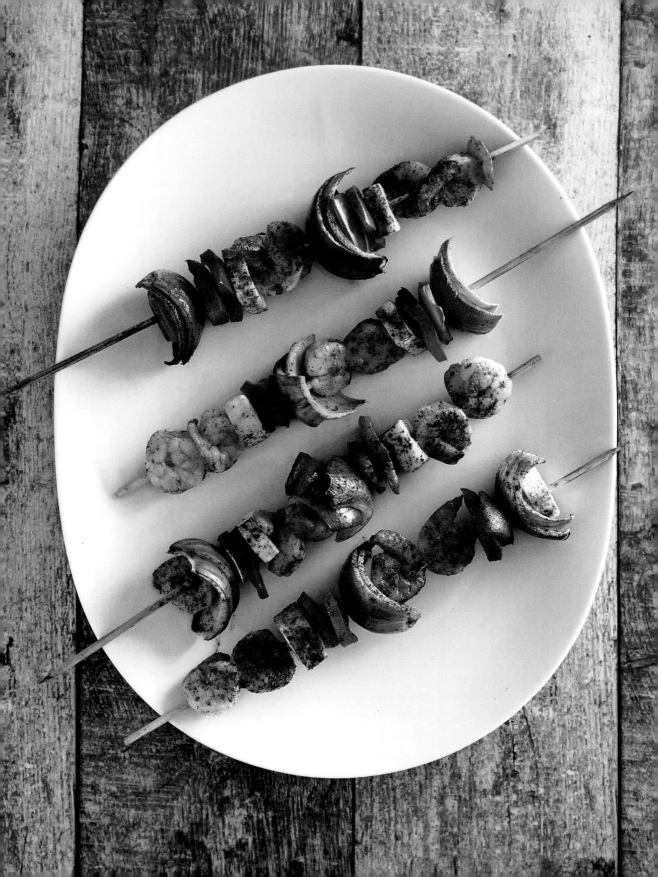

Shrimp Kebabs

Everyone loves kebabs, but it's not always barbecue weather outside. The air fryer makes these supersimple and crispy like the grill in no time! You can customize it with your favorite flavors and veggies and even brush with a sugar-free barbecue sauce for an extra kick!

- **Hands-On Time: 10 minutes**
- **Cook Time: 7 minutes**

Serves 2

18 medium shelled and deveined shrimp

1 medium zucchini, cut into 1" cubes

½ medium red bell pepper, cut into 1"-thick squares

¼ medium red onion, cut into 1"-thick squares

1½ tablespoons coconut oil, melted

2 teaspoons chili powder

½ teaspoon paprika

¼ teaspoon ground black pepper

1 Soak four 6" bamboo skewers in water for 30 minutes. Place a shrimp on the skewer, then a zucchini, a pepper, and an onion. Repeat until all ingredients are utilized.

2 Brush each kebab with coconut oil. Sprinkle with chili powder, paprika, and black pepper. Place kebabs into the air fryer basket.

3 Adjust the temperature to 400°F and set the timer for 7 minutes or until shrimp is fully cooked and veggies are tender.

4 Flip kebabs halfway through the cooking time. Serve warm.

PER SERVING

CALORIES: 166	FAT: 10.7 g
PROTEIN: 9.5 g	SODIUM: 391 mg
FIBER: 3.1 g	CARBOHYDRATES: 8.5 g
NET CARBOHYDRATES: 5.4 g	SUGAR: 4.5 g

Simple Buttery Cod

This is a delicious and simple recipe that's a perfect weeknight staple. To make sure this dish is full of buttery flavor, buy a quality butter. Irish butter, such as Kerrygold, is deeper in color and has a much richer flavor than a store-brand butter.

- **Hands-On Time: 5 minutes**
- **Cook Time: 8 minutes**

Serves 2

2 (4-ounce) cod fillets

2 tablespoons salted butter, melted

1 teaspoon Old Bay seasoning

½ medium lemon, sliced

1 Place cod fillets into a 6″ round baking dish. Brush each fillet with butter and sprinkle with Old Bay seasoning. Lay two lemon slices on each fillet. Cover the dish with foil and place into the air fryer basket.

2 Adjust the temperature to 350°F and set the timer for 8 minutes.

3 Flip halfway through the cooking time. When cooked, internal temperature should be at least 145°F. Serve warm.

PER SERVING

CALORIES: 179	**FAT:** 11.1 g
PROTEIN: 17.4 g	**SODIUM:** 714 mg
FIBER: 0.0 g	**CARBOHYDRATES:** 0.0 g
NET CARBOHYDRATES: 0.0 g	**SUGAR:** 0.0 g

Vegetarian Main Dishes

Even though meats are an easy way to get the protein essential for a healthy ketogenic diet, vegetables are also really important to making sure you're properly nourished. And the air fryer is definitely intended for more than cooking meats! These vegetarian main dishes are great for if you're trying out a Meatless Monday or simply getting your protein from another source than meat.

Loaded Cauliflower Steak

Cauliflower steaks are a great vegetarian option that have nutrients and flavor. Roasting them with buffalo sauce gives you a light and spicy dish that is totally guilt-free! Serve with crumbled blue cheese or ranch dressing if you need to tone down the spice!

- **Hands-On Time: 5 minutes**
- **Cook Time: 7 minutes**

Serves 4

1 medium head cauliflower
¼ cup hot sauce
2 tablespoons salted butter, melted
¼ cup blue cheese crumbles
¼ cup full-fat ranch dressing

1 Remove cauliflower leaves. Slice the head in ½"-thick slices.

2 In a small bowl, mix hot sauce and butter. Brush the mixture over the cauliflower.

3 Place each cauliflower steak into the air fryer, working in batches if necessary.

4 Adjust the temperature to 400°F and set the timer for 7 minutes.

5 When cooked, edges will begin turning dark and caramelized.

6 To serve, sprinkle steaks with crumbled blue cheese. Drizzle with ranch dressing.

PER SERVING

CALORIES: 122
PROTEIN: 4.9 g
FIBER: 3.0 g
NET CARBOHYDRATES: 4.7 g

FAT: 8.4 g
SODIUM: 283 mg
CARBOHYDRATES: 7.7 g
SUGAR: 2.9 g

Three-Cheese Zucchini Boats

Zucchini is a low-carb vegetable that is high in water content, which means it helps keep you fuller longer, discouraging overeating. This cheesy, handheld dish gives you all of those benefits, plus a nice crunch in each bite that you won't find in many low-carb meals!

- **Hands-On Time: 15 minutes**
- **Cook Time: 20 minutes**

Serves 2

2 medium zucchini

1 tablespoon avocado oil

¼ cup low-carb, no-sugar-added pasta sauce

¼ cup full-fat ricotta cheese

¼ cup shredded mozzarella cheese

¼ teaspoon dried oregano

¼ teaspoon garlic powder

½ teaspoon dried parsley

2 tablespoons grated vegetarian Parmesan cheese

1 Cut off 1" from the top and bottom of each zucchini. Slice zucchini in half lengthwise and use a spoon to scoop out a bit of the inside, making room for filling. Brush with oil and spoon 2 tablespoons pasta sauce into each shell.

2 In a medium bowl, mix ricotta, mozzarella, oregano, garlic powder, and parsley. Spoon the mixture into each zucchini shell. Place stuffed zucchini shells into the air fryer basket.

3 Adjust the temperature to 350°F and set the timer for 20 minutes.

4 To remove from the fryer basket, use tongs or a spatula and carefully lift out. Top with Parmesan. Serve immediately.

PER SERVING

CALORIES: 215	**FAT:** 14.9 g
PROTEIN: 10.5 g	**SODIUM:** 386 mg
FIBER: 2.7 g	**CARBOHYDRATES:** 9.3 g
NET CARBOHYDRATES: 6.6 g	**SUGAR:** 5.2 g

Portobello Mini Pizzas

This low-calorie alternative to a low-carb pizza really hits the spot! You won't miss out on an ounce of flavor, plus portobello mushrooms are rich in B vitamins that help maintain healthy skin, hair, and eyes!

- **Hands-On Time: 10 minutes**
- **Cook Time: 10 minutes**

Serves 2

2 large portobello mushrooms

2 tablespoons unsalted butter, melted

½ teaspoon garlic powder

⅔ cup shredded mozzarella cheese

4 grape tomatoes, sliced

2 leaves fresh basil, chopped

1 tablespoon balsamic vinegar

1 Scoop out the inside of the mushrooms, leaving just the caps. Brush each cap with butter and sprinkle with garlic powder.

2 Fill each cap with mozzarella and sliced tomatoes. Place each mini pizza into a 6″ round baking pan. Place pan into the air fryer basket.

3 Adjust the temperature to 380°F and set the timer for 10 minutes.

4 Carefully remove the pizzas from the fryer basket and garnish with basil and a drizzle of vinegar.

PER SERVING

CALORIES: 244	**FAT:** 18.5 g
PROTEIN: 10.4 g	**SODIUM:** 244 mg
FIBER: 1.4 g	**CARBOHYDRATES:** 6.8 g
NET CARBOHYDRATES: 5.4 g	**SUGAR:** 4.3 g

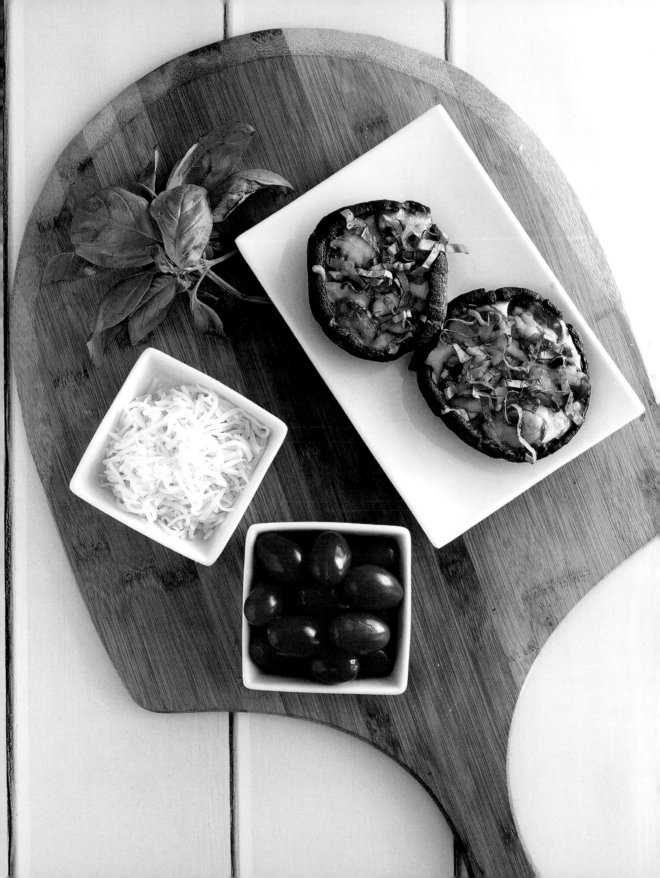

Veggie Quesadilla

This dish uses a simple flatbread instead of a traditional low-carb tortilla. Low-carb tortillas often contain wheat, gluten, and high amounts of fiber, which for some people may cause bloating, weight gain, and trigger an insulin response. This sautéed veggie-filled alternative is so filling and full of nutrients you won't even miss traditional quesadillas.

- **Hands-On Time: 10 minutes**
- **Cook Time: 5 minutes**

Serves 2

1 tablespoon coconut oil

½ medium green bell pepper, seeded and chopped

¼ cup diced red onion

¼ cup chopped white mushrooms

4 flatbread dough tortillas

⅔ cup shredded pepper jack cheese

½ medium avocado, peeled, pitted, and mashed

¼ cup full-fat sour cream

¼ cup mild salsa

ALTERNATIVE TORTILLAS
Though some people choose to avoid wheat and gluten while following a ketogenic diet, others find that low-carb tortillas are a helpful staple. Pork rind tortillas are lower in carbs than wheat tortillas and a boost of protein. As an alternative look for 100 percent flax tortillas or wraps made from turmeric.

1. In a medium skillet over medium heat, warm coconut oil. Add pepper, onion, and mushrooms to skillet and sauté until peppers begin to soften, 3–5 minutes.

2. Place two tortillas on a work surface and sprinkle each with half of cheese. Top with sautéed veggies, sprinkle with remaining cheese, and place remaining two tortillas on top. Place quesadillas carefully into the air fryer basket.

3. Adjust the temperature to 400°F and set the timer for 5 minutes.

4. Flip the quesadillas halfway through the cooking time. Serve warm with avocado, sour cream, and salsa.

PER SERVING

CALORIES: 795	**FAT:** 61.3 g
PROTEIN: 34.5 g	**SODIUM:** 1,051 mg
FIBER: 6.5 g	**CARBOHYDRATES:** 19.4 g
NET CARBOHYDRATES: 12.9 g	**SUGAR:** 7.4 g

Roasted Veggie Bowl

Vegetables are a very important part of a keto diet. Equally important is deciding which vegetables to eat. This bowl is made up of a combination of very low-carb and high-fiber veggies to feed your body tons of nutrients while satisfying your palate.

- **Hands-On Time: 10 minutes**
- **Cook Time: 15 minutes**

Serves 2

1 cup broccoli florets

1 cup quartered Brussels sprouts

½ cup cauliflower florets

¼ medium white onion, peeled and sliced ¼" thick

½ medium green bell pepper, seeded and sliced ¼" thick

1 tablespoon coconut oil

2 teaspoons chili powder

½ teaspoon garlic powder

½ teaspoon cumin

1 Toss all ingredients together in a large bowl until vegetables are fully coated with oil and seasoning.

2 Pour vegetables into the air fryer basket.

3 Adjust the temperature to 360°F and set the timer for 15 minutes.

4 Shake two or three times during cooking. Serve warm.

PER SERVING

CALORIES: 121	FAT: 7.1 g
PROTEIN: 4.3 g	SODIUM: 112 mg
FIBER: 5.2 g	CARBOHYDRATES: 13.1 g
NET CARBOHYDRATES: 7.9 g	SUGAR: 3.8 g

MAKE IT A MEAL!

To make this an even more filling meal, add a serving of sautéed cauliflower rice to your bowl. Simply buy a steamer bag of riced or pearled cauliflower, follow package instructions, add butter with seasonings, and top it with your roasted veggies.

Spinach Artichoke Casserole

This casserole boosts one of your favorite dips to the next level. With the same warm creaminess, but with more nutrients and substance than the original dip, you'll be happy to make this meatless meal a part of your regular rotation!

- **Hands-On Time: 15 minutes**
- **Cook Time: 15 minutes**

Serves 4

1 tablespoon salted butter, melted

¼ cup diced yellow onion

8 ounces full-fat cream cheese, softened

⅓ cup full-fat mayonnaise

⅓ cup full-fat sour cream

¼ cup chopped pickled jalapeños

2 cups fresh spinach, chopped

2 cups cauliflower florets, chopped

1 cup artichoke hearts, chopped

1 In a large bowl, mix butter, onion, cream cheese, mayonnaise, and sour cream. Fold in jalapeños, spinach, cauliflower, and artichokes.

2 Pour the mixture into a 4-cup round baking dish. Cover with foil and place into the air fryer basket.

3 Adjust the temperature to 370°F and set the timer for 15 minutes.

4 In the last 2 minutes of cooking, remove the foil to brown the top. Serve warm.

PER SERVING

CALORIES: 423	FAT: 36.3 g
PROTEIN: 6.7 g	SODIUM: 495 mg
FIBER: 5.3 g	CARBOHYDRATES: 12.1 g
NET CARBOHYDRATES: 6.8 g	SUGAR: 4.4 g

Cheesy Zoodle Bake

This is a dish the whole family will love! The spiralized zucchini tossed in two different types of cheese make this a gooey and delicious and filling meal.

- **Hands-On Time: 10 minutes**
- **Cook Time: 8 minutes**

Serves 4

2 tablespoons salted butter
¼ cup diced white onion
½ teaspoon minced garlic
½ cup heavy whipping cream
2 ounces full-fat cream
 cheese
1 cup shredded sharp
 Cheddar cheese
2 medium zucchini, spiralized

CRUNCHY TOP

To get that classic browned top that many casseroles have, add cheese crisps to top. These can be found in your local grocery store or made by baking a thin layer of shredded cheese for just a few minutes. Broil for 3–5 minutes until the cheese gets golden and crispy.

1 In a large saucepan over medium heat, melt butter. Add onion and sauté until it begins to soften, 1–3 minutes. Add garlic and sauté 30 seconds, then pour in cream and add cream cheese.

2 Remove the pan from heat and stir in Cheddar. Add the zucchini and toss in the sauce, then put into a 4-cup round baking dish. Cover the dish with foil and place into the air fryer basket.

3 Adjust the temperature to 370°F and set the timer for 8 minutes.

4 After 6 minutes remove the foil and let the top brown for remaining cooking time. Stir and serve.

PER SERVING

CALORIES: 337	**FAT:** 28.4 g
PROTEIN: 9.6 g	**SODIUM:** 298 mg
FIBER: 1.2 g	**CARBOHYDRATES:** 5.9 g
NET CARBOHYDRATES: 4.7 g	**SUGAR:** 4.3 g

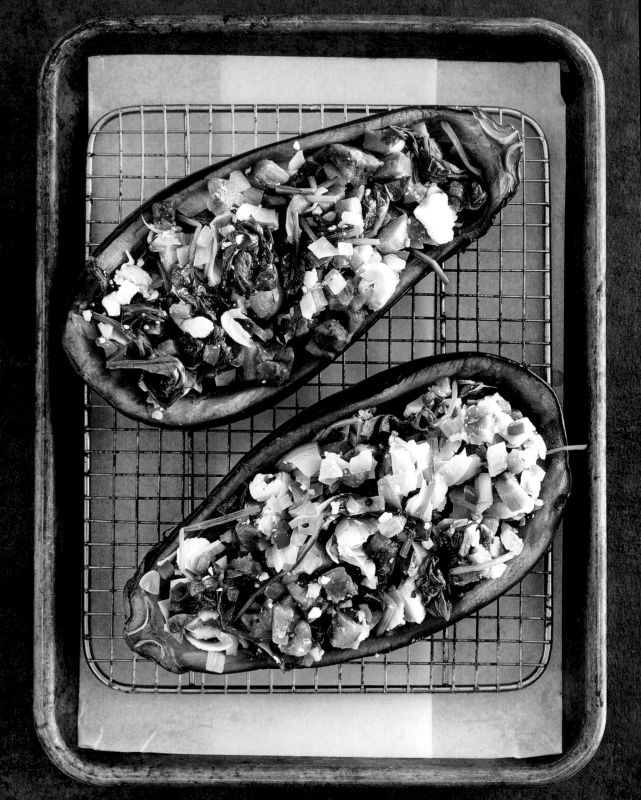

Greek Stuffed Eggplant

Perfectly roasted and filled with nutrient-rich veggies, stuffed eggplant is a perfect fresh and fibrous meal even if you're not vegetarian! This meatless masterpiece is bursting with succulent Greek flavors to keep you satisfied!

- **Hands-On Time: 15 minutes**
- **Cook Time: 20 minutes**

Serves 2

1 large eggplant

2 tablespoons unsalted butter

¼ medium yellow onion, diced

¼ cup chopped artichoke hearts

1 cup fresh spinach

2 tablespoons diced red bell pepper

½ cup crumbled feta

1 Slice eggplant in half lengthwise and scoop out flesh, leaving enough inside for shell to remain intact. Take eggplant that was scooped out, chop it, and set aside.

2 In a medium skillet over medium heat, add butter and onion. Sauté until onions begin to soften, about 3–5 minutes. Add chopped eggplant, artichokes, spinach, and bell pepper. Continue cooking 5 minutes until peppers soften and spinach wilts. Remove from the heat and gently fold in the feta.

3 Place filling into each eggplant shell and place into the air fryer basket.

4 Adjust the temperature to 320°F and set the timer for 20 minutes.

5 Eggplant will be tender when done. Serve warm.

PER SERVING

CALORIES: 291	FAT: 18.7 g
PROTEIN: 9.4 g	SODIUM: 374 mg
FIBER: 10.8 g	CARBOHYDRATES: 22.6 g
NET CARBOHYDRATES: 11.8 g	SUGAR: 12.5 g

Roasted Broccoli Salad

Broccoli takes on a different taste when roasted, and in this salad it creates the perfect hint of sweet. The almonds add a nice crunch for contrast, not to mention a burst of healthy fats. Almonds are a great addition to salads and taste even better when roasted. You can even roast almonds in the air fryer while you prepare a meal (see Ranch Roasted Almonds in Chapter 3)!

- **Hands-On Time: 10 minutes**
- **Cook Time: 7 minutes**

Serves 2

3 cups fresh broccoli florets

2 tablespoons salted butter, melted

¼ cup sliced almonds

½ medium lemon

1 Place broccoli into a 6″ round baking dish. Pour butter over broccoli. Add almonds and toss. Place dish into the air fryer basket.

2 Adjust the temperature to 380°F and set the timer for 7 minutes.

3 Stir halfway through the cooking time.

4 When timer beeps, zest lemon onto broccoli and squeeze juice into pan. Toss. Serve warm.

PER SERVING

CALORIES: 215	FAT: 16.3 g	
PROTEIN: 6.4 g	SODIUM: 136 mg	
FIBER: 5.0 g	CARBOHYDRATES: 12.1 g	
NET CARBOHYDRATES: 7.1 g	SUGAR: 3.0 g	

Whole Roasted Lemon Cauliflower

This is a bright and refreshing entrée with plenty of substance for a meal, or in smaller portions it can be served as a nutritious side dish with just the right amount of tang. The options for dressing up cauliflower are endless, and this recipe proves it.

- **Hands-On Time: 5 minutes**
- **Cook Time: 15 minutes**

Serves 4

1 medium head cauliflower
2 tablespoons salted butter, melted
1 medium lemon
½ teaspoon garlic powder
1 teaspoon dried parsley

1 Remove the leaves from the head of cauliflower and brush it with melted butter. Cut the lemon in half and zest one half onto the cauliflower. Squeeze the juice of the zested lemon half and pour it over the cauliflower.

2 Sprinkle with garlic powder and parsley. Place cauliflower head into the air fryer basket.

3 Adjust the temperature to 350°F and set the timer for 15 minutes.

4 Check cauliflower every 5 minutes to avoid overcooking. It should be fork tender.

5 To serve, squeeze juice from other lemon half over cauliflower. Serve immediately.

PER SERVING

CALORIES: 91
PROTEIN: 3.0 g
FIBER: 3.2 g
NET CARBOHYDRATES: 5.2 g

FAT: 5.7 g
SODIUM: 90 mg
CARBOHYDRATES: 8.4 g
SUGAR: 3.1 g

Cheesy Cauliflower Pizza Crust

Cauliflower pizza crust is a trendy alternative to regular crust, and for a good reason! It's full of nutrients and tastes amazing! Load this pizza up with cheese and even your favorite low-carb veggies for a fresh and filling vegetarian meal!

- **Hands-On Time: 15 minutes**
- **Cook Time: 11 minutes**

Serves 2

1 (12-ounce) steamer bag cauliflower
½ cup shredded sharp Cheddar cheese
1 large egg
2 tablespoons blanched finely ground almond flour
1 teaspoon Italian blend seasoning

HOMEMADE IS BETTER!

Homemade cauliflower pizza crust is always better than store-bought versions! Often, brands will use additives like potato starch to make their pizza crusts firmer and more shelf stable. These tricky fillers can add loads of unnecessary carbs!

1 Cook cauliflower according to package instructions. Remove from bag and place into cheesecloth or paper towel to remove excess water. Place cauliflower into a large bowl.

2 Add cheese, egg, almond flour, and Italian seasoning to the bowl and mix well.

3 Cut a piece of parchment to fit your air fryer basket. Press cauliflower into 6" round circle. Place into the air fryer basket.

4 Adjust the temperature to 360°F and set the timer for 11 minutes.

5 After 7 minutes, flip the pizza crust.

6 Add preferred toppings to pizza. Place back into air fryer basket and cook an additional 4 minutes or until fully cooked and golden. Serve immediately.

PER SERVING

CALORIES: 230	**FAT:** 14.2 g
PROTEIN: 14.9 g	**SODIUM:** 257 mg
FIBER: 4.7 g	**CARBOHYDRATES:** 10.0 g
NET CARBOHYDRATES: 5.3 g	**SUGAR:** 4.2 g

Quiche-Stuffed Peppers

Add some excitement to your crustless quiche by baking it right in a pepper! These easy quiches will help you get more vegetables in your day, and there's no limit to the different ways you can customize them!

- **Hands-On Time: 5 minutes**
- **Cook Time: 15 minutes**

Serves 2

2 medium green bell peppers
3 large eggs
¼ cup full-fat ricotta cheese
¼ cup diced yellow onion
½ cup chopped broccoli
½ cup shredded medium
   Cheddar cheese

1 Cut the tops off of the peppers and remove the seeds and white membranes with a small knife.

2 In a medium bowl, whisk eggs and ricotta.

3 Add onion and broccoli. Pour the egg and vegetable mixture evenly into each pepper. Top with Cheddar. Place peppers into a 4-cup round baking dish and place into the air fryer basket.

4 Adjust the temperature to 350°F and set the timer for 15 minutes.

5 Eggs will be mostly firm and peppers tender when fully cooked. Serve immediately.

PER SERVING

CALORIES: 314	**FAT:** 18.7 g
PROTEIN: 21.6 g	**SODIUM:** 325 mg
FIBER: 3.0 g	**CARBOHYDRATES:** 10.8 g
NET CARBOHYDRATES: 7.8 g	**SUGAR:** 4.5 g

Roasted Garlic White Zucchini Rolls

This recipe turns those lasagna layers into perfectly portioned zucchini rolls! It also swaps out the meat for mushrooms, resulting in a lower-calorie dish.

- **Hands-On Time: 20 minutes**
- **Cook Time: 20 minutes**

Serves 4

2 medium zucchini

2 tablespoons unsalted butter

¼ white onion, peeled and diced

½ teaspoon finely minced roasted garlic

¼ cup heavy cream

2 tablespoons vegetable broth

⅛ teaspoon xanthan gum

½ cup full-fat ricotta cheese

¼ teaspoon salt

½ teaspoon garlic powder

¼ teaspoon dried oregano

2 cups spinach, chopped

½ cup sliced baby portobello mushrooms

¾ cup shredded mozzarella cheese, divided

WHY XANTHAN GUM?

Xanthan gum is a thickener that is often used in ketogenic cooking. It doesn't change the flavor, but it helps create a thicker, more traditional sauce.

1 Using a mandoline or sharp knife, slice zucchini into long strips lengthwise. Place strips between paper towels to absorb moisture. Set aside.

2 In a medium saucepan over medium heat, melt butter. Add onion and sauté until fragrant. Add garlic and sauté 30 seconds.

3 Pour in heavy cream, broth, and xanthan gum. Turn off heat and whisk mixture until it begins to thicken, about 3 minutes.

4 In a medium bowl, add ricotta, salt, garlic powder, and oregano and mix well. Fold in spinach, mushrooms, and ½ cup mozzarella.

5 Pour half of the sauce into a 6" round baking pan. To assemble the rolls, place two strips of zucchini on a work surface. Spoon 2 tablespoons of ricotta mixture onto the slices and roll up. Place seam side down on top of sauce. Repeat with remaining ingredients.

6 Pour remaining sauce over the rolls and sprinkle with remaining mozzarella. Cover with foil and place into the air fryer basket.

7 Adjust the temperature to 350°F and set the timer for 20 minutes.

8 In the last 5 minutes, remove the foil to brown the cheese. Serve immediately.

PER SERVING

CALORIES: 245	**FAT:** 18.9 g
PROTEIN: 10.5 g	**SODIUM:** 346 mg
FIBER: 1.8 g	**CARBOHYDRATES:** 7.1 g
NET CARBOHYDRATES: 5.3 g	**SUGAR:** 3.8 g

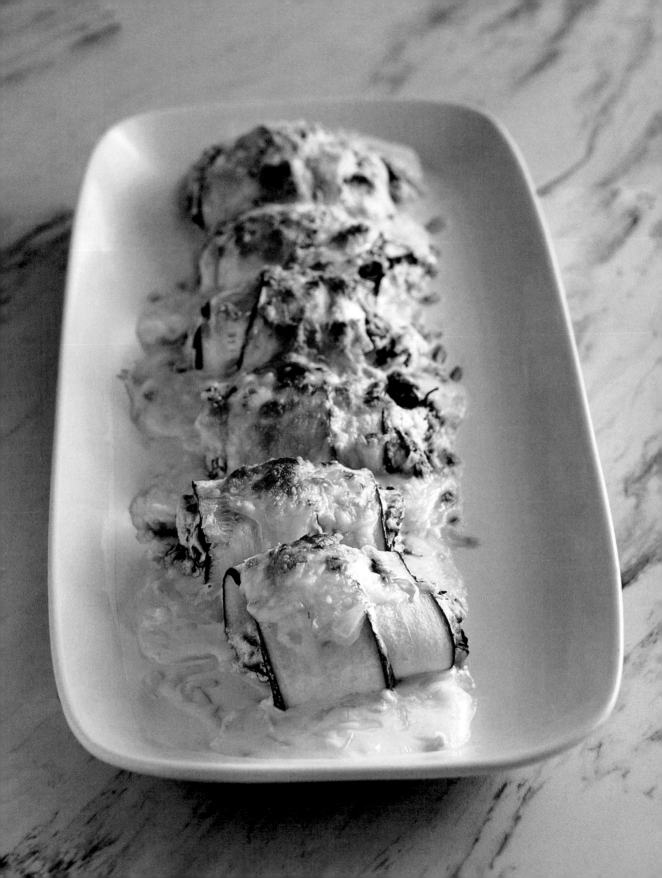

Spicy Parmesan Artichokes

Artichokes are a versatile food that are rich in vitamin B_{12}, which helps maintain the health of nerve cells as well as aiding in digestion and heart health. They bake perfectly in your air fryer, and with just a bit of cheese and seasoning they're transformed into an absolutely delicious dish!

- **Hands-On Time: 10 minutes**
- **Cook Time: 10 minutes**

Serves 4

2 medium artichokes, trimmed and quartered, center removed

2 tablespoons coconut oil

1 large egg, beaten

½ cup grated vegetarian Parmesan cheese

¼ cup blanched finely ground almond flour

½ teaspoon crushed red pepper flakes

1   In a large bowl, toss artichokes in coconut oil and then dip each piece into the egg.

2   Mix the Parmesan and almond flour in a large bowl. Add artichoke pieces and toss to cover as completely as possible, sprinkle with pepper flakes. Place into the air fryer basket.

3   Adjust the temperature to 400°F and set the timer for 10 minutes.

4   Toss the basket two times during cooking. Serve warm.

PER SERVING

CALORIES: 189

PROTEIN: 7.9 g

FIBER: 4.2 g

NET CARBOHYDRATES: 5.8 g

FAT: 13.5 g

SODIUM: 294 mg

CARBOHYDRATES: 10.0 g

SUGAR: 0.9 g

Zucchini Cauliflower Fritters

These fritters are a crispy way to make sure your kids are getting their vegetables! Your air fryer gives them a crispy outside and a flavor-filled middle, meaning sinking your teeth into them will always put a smile on your face! For a nice creamy addition, scoop a dollop of full-fat sour cream on top!

- **Hands-On Time: 15 minutes**
- **Cook Time: 12 minutes**

Serves 2

1 (12-ounce) cauliflower steamer bag
1 medium zucchini, shredded
¼ cup almond flour
1 large egg
½ teaspoon garlic powder
¼ cup grated vegetarian Parmesan cheese

1 Cook cauliflower according to package instructions and drain excess moisture in cheesecloth or paper towel. Place into a large bowl.

2 Place zucchini into paper towel and pat down to remove excess moisture. Add to bowl with cauliflower. Add remaining ingredients.

3 Divide the mixture evenly and form four patties. Press into ¼"-thick patties. Place each into the air fryer basket.

4 Adjust the temperature to 320°F and set the timer for 12 minutes.

5 Fritters will be firm when fully cooked. Allow to cool 5 minutes before moving. Serve warm.

PER SERVING

CALORIES: 217	FAT: 12.0 g
PROTEIN: 13.7 g	SODIUM: 263 mg
FIBER: 6.5 g	CARBOHYDRATES: 16.1 g
NET CARBOHYDRATES: 8.5 g	SUGAR: 6.8 g

Basic Spaghetti Squash

Spaghetti squash can be used to create a wide variety of dishes from savory Italian dinners to breakfast boats. Your air fryer can help you get the perfect bake on your squash, and you'll be on your way to enjoying all of its versatile qualities in no time!

- **Hands-On Time: 10 minutes**
- **Cook Time: 45 minutes**

Serves 2

½ large spaghetti squash

1 tablespoon coconut oil

2 tablespoons salted butter, melted

½ teaspoon garlic powder

1 teaspoon dried parsley

PAIR WITH NO-SUGAR-ADDED TOMATO SAUCE

This spaghetti squash is great served with tomato sauce, but when you are out shopping for sauce be cautious and read labels. Many tomato pasta sauces have added sugars to make the sauce sweet. Tomatoes naturally have carbs, but try to avoid sauces that specifically add sugar for taste. There are low-carb-friendly options out there, like Rao's marinara, which has only 4 grams net carbs per serving. If you can't find them in the pasta aisle, try looking in the health food section for better options.

1   Brush shell of spaghetti squash with coconut oil. Place the skin side down and brush the inside with butter. Sprinkle with garlic powder and parsley.

2   Place squash with the skin side down into the air fryer basket.

3   Adjust the temperature to 350°F and set the timer for 30 minutes.

4   When the timer beeps, flip the squash so skin side is up and cook an additional 15 minutes or until fork tender. Serve warm.

PER SERVING

CALORIES: 182		**FAT:** 11.7 g	
PROTEIN: 1.9 g		**SODIUM:** 134 mg	
FIBER: 3.9 g		**CARBOHYDRATES:** 18.2 g	
NET CARBOHYDRATES: 14.3 g		**SUGAR:** 7.0 g	

Spaghetti Squash Alfredo

Spaghetti squash is a great alternative to regular pasta. It's right there in the name! Especially if you're someone who cares about texture, you'll love this smart swap and all the yummy Alfredo sauce it's baked in!

- **Hands-On Time: 10 minutes**
- **Cook Time: 15 minutes**

Serves 2

½ large cooked spaghetti squash

2 tablespoons salted butter, melted

½ cup low-carb Alfredo sauce

¼ cup grated vegetarian Parmesan cheese

½ teaspoon garlic powder

1 teaspoon dried parsley

¼ teaspoon ground peppercorn

½ cup shredded Italian blend cheese

1 Using a fork, remove the strands of spaghetti squash from the shell. Place into a large bowl with butter and Alfredo sauce. Sprinkle with Parmesan, garlic powder, parsley, and peppercorn.

2 Pour into a 4-cup round baking dish and top with shredded cheese. Place dish into the air fryer basket.

3 Adjust the temperature to 320°F and set the timer for 15 minutes.

4 When finished, cheese will be golden and bubbling. Serve immediately.

PER SERVING

CALORIES: 375	FAT: 24.2 g
PROTEIN: 13.5 g	SODIUM: 950 mg
FIBER: 4.0 g	CARBOHYDRATES: 24.1 g
NET CARBOHYDRATES: 20.1 g	SUGAR: 8.0 g

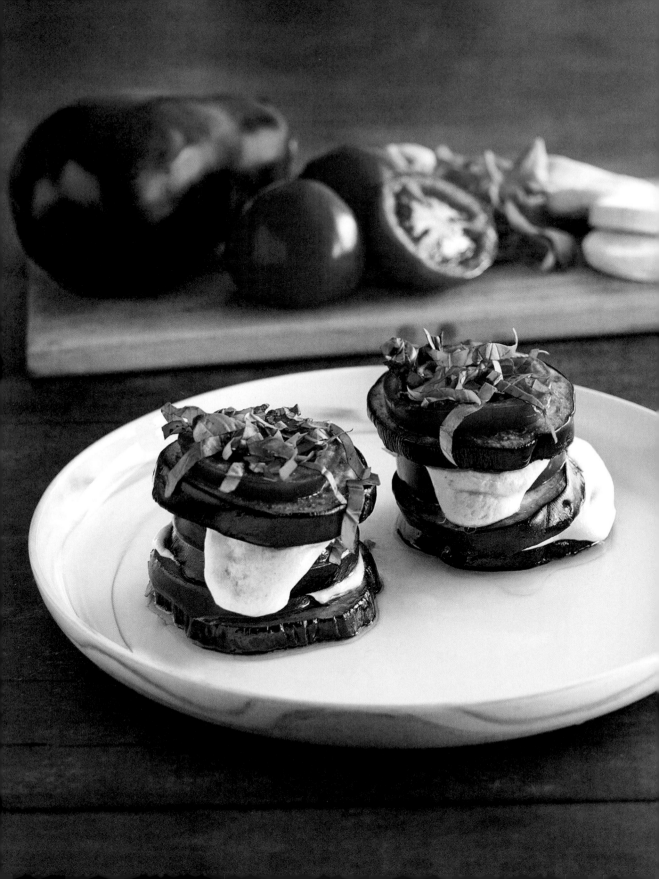

Caprese Eggplant Stacks

These stacks are a warm twist on the classic fresh caprese salad.

- **Hands-On Time: 5 minutes**
- **Cook Time: 12 minutes**

Serves 4

1 medium eggplant, cut into ¼″ slices

2 large tomatoes, cut into ¼″ slices

4 ounces fresh mozzarella, cut into ½-ounce slices

2 tablespoons olive oil

¼ cup fresh basil, sliced

1 In a 6″ round baking dish, place four slices of eggplant on the bottom. Place a slice of tomato on top of each eggplant round, then mozzarella, then eggplant. Repeat as necessary.

2 Drizzle with olive oil. Cover dish with foil and place dish into the air fryer basket.

3 Adjust the temperature to 350°F and set the timer for 12 minutes.

4 When done, eggplant will be tender. Garnish with fresh basil to serve.

PER SERVING

CALORIES: 195	FAT: 12.7 g
PROTEIN: 8.5 g	SODIUM: 184 mg
FIBER: 5.2 g	CARBOHYDRATES: 12.7 g
NET CARBOHYDRATES: 7.5 g	SUGAR: 7.5 g

Crustless Spinach Cheese Pie

This creamy and savory pie is a great light lunch that you won't be able to get enough of!

- **Hands-On Time: 10 minutes**
- **Cook Time: 20 minutes**

Serves 4

6 large eggs

¼ cup heavy whipping cream

1 cup frozen chopped spinach, drained

1 cup shredded sharp Cheddar cheese

¼ cup diced yellow onion

1 In a medium bowl, whisk eggs and add cream. Add remaining ingredients to bowl.

2 Pour into a 6″ round baking dish. Place into the air fryer basket.

3 Adjust the temperature to 320°F and set the timer for 20 minutes.

4 Eggs will be firm and slightly browned when cooked. Serve immediately.

PER SERVING

CALORIES: 288	FAT: 20.0 g
PROTEIN: 18.0 g	SODIUM: 322 mg
FIBER: 1.3 g	CARBOHYDRATES: 3.9 g
NET CARBOHYDRATES: 2.6 g	SUGAR: 1.5 g

Broccoli Crust Pizza

Rich with vitamins, fiber, and phytonutrients, broccoli is a great option for your keto diet. Making it into a pizza crust is a fun and unique spin to make sure you, or your kiddos, are getting their veggies in while enjoying something supertasty!

- **Hands-On Time: 15 minutes**
- **Cook Time: 12 minutes**

Serves 4

3 cups riced broccoli, steamed and drained well

1 large egg

½ cup grated vegetarian Parmesan cheese

3 tablespoons low-carb Alfredo sauce

½ cup shredded mozzarella cheese

1   In a large bowl, mix broccoli, egg, and Parmesan.

2   Cut a piece of parchment to fit your air fryer basket. Press out the pizza mixture to fit on the parchment, working in two batches if necessary. Place into the air fryer basket.

3   Adjust the temperature to 370°F and set the timer for 5 minutes.

4   When the timer beeps, the crust should be firm enough to flip. If not, add 2 additional minutes. Flip crust.

5   Top with Alfredo sauce and mozzarella. Return to the air fryer basket and cook an additional 7 minutes or until cheese is golden and bubbling. Serve warm.

PER SERVING

CALORIES: 136	FAT: 7.6 g
PROTEIN: 9.9 g	SODIUM: 421 mg
FIBER: 2.3 g	CARBOHYDRATES: 5.7 g
NET CARBOHYDRATES: 3.4 g	SUGAR: 1.1 g

Italian Baked Egg and Veggies

One concern for people who follow a vegetarian and a keto diet is if they're getting enough protein. If you're doing keto for weight loss, making sure you hit your protein macronutrient goal is a great way to prevent muscle loss, and eggs are an excellent meatless source of protein. This recipe pairs the egg with nutrient-rich veggies as well as delicious seasoning to round out the entrée.

- **Hands-On Time: 10 minutes**
- **Cook Time: 10 minutes**

Serves 2

2 tablespoons salted butter

1 small zucchini, sliced lengthwise and quartered

½ medium green bell pepper, seeded and diced

1 cup fresh spinach, chopped

1 medium Roma tomato, diced

2 large eggs

¼ teaspoon onion powder

¼ teaspoon garlic powder

½ teaspoon dried basil

¼ teaspoon dried oregano

1 Grease two (4") ramekins with 1 tablespoon butter each.

2 In a large bowl, toss zucchini, bell pepper, spinach, and tomatoes. Divide the mixture in two and place half in each ramekin.

3 Crack an egg on top of each ramekin and sprinkle with onion powder, garlic powder, basil, and oregano. Place into the air fryer basket.

4 Adjust the temperature to 330°F and set the timer for 10 minutes.

5 Serve immediately.

PER SERVING

CALORIES: 150	**FAT:** 10.0 g
PROTEIN: 8.3 g	**SODIUM:** 135 mg
FIBER: 2.2 g	**CARBOHYDRATES:** 6.6 g
NET CARBOHYDRATES: 4.4 g	**SUGAR:** 3.7 g

BBQ "Pulled" Mushrooms

Get a similar taste and texture to barbecue pulled pork with this unique swap. Mushrooms are a great substitute for meat because they have a real substance to them. By "pulling" the mushrooms and giving them a quick air fryer bake with sauce, you have a surprisingly delightful vegetarian dish!

- **Hands-On Time: 5 minutes**
- **Cook Time: 12 minutes**

Serves 2

4 large portobello
    mushrooms

1 tablespoon salted butter,
    melted

¼ teaspoon ground black
    pepper

1 teaspoon chili powder

1 teaspoon paprika

¼ teaspoon onion powder

½ cup low-carb, sugar-free
    barbecue sauce

LOW-CARB BARBECUE SAUCE

Just like with ketchup, most premade barbecue sauces are loaded with sugar! Always be sure to read the nutritional labels to make sure you're opting for sauces with the fewest ingredients possible so you can avoid hidden carbs or fillers.

1 Remove stem and scoop out the underside of each mushroom. Brush the caps with butter and sprinkle with pepper, chili powder, paprika, and onion powder.

2 Place mushrooms into the air fryer basket.

3 Adjust the temperature to 400°F and set the timer for 8 minutes.

4 When the timer beeps, remove mushrooms from the basket and place on a cutting board or work surface. Using two forks, gently pull the mushrooms apart, creating strands.

5 Place mushroom strands into a 4-cup round baking dish with barbecue sauce. Place dish into the air fryer basket.

6 Adjust the temperature to 350°F and set the timer for 4 minutes.

7 Stir halfway through the cooking time. Serve warm.

PER SERVING

CALORIES: 108	**FAT:** 5.9 g
PROTEIN: 3.3 g	**SODIUM:** 476 mg
FIBER: 2.7 g	**CARBOHYDRATES:** 10.9 g
NET CARBOHYDRATES: 8.2 g	**SUGAR:** 3.6 g

9

Desserts

Desserts are usually the toughest thing for anybody to give up on any kind of diet. Thankfully, there are a ton of keto-friendly options to keep you on track while keeping your sweet tooth satisfied! With your air fryer, you're able to create a wide range of perfectly portioned goodies that always hit the spot! As an added bonus, with the smaller cooking chamber than a traditional oven, these treats will also cook in practically no time! From Chocolate Espresso Mini Cheesecake to Caramel Monkey Bread, this chapter has enough sweet treats to make sure you never feel deprived!

Almond Butter Cookie Balls

These cookie balls are a poppable version of a warm and gooey chocolate chip cookie! Be sure to use an almond butter that has two ingredients maximum (almonds and salt); many brands enhance the flavor with ingredients like sugar and honey, adding a ton of carbs you don't need.

- **Hands-On Time: 5 minutes**
- **Cook Time: 10 minutes**

Yields 10 balls (1 ball per serving)

1 cup almond butter

1 large egg

1 teaspoon vanilla extract

¼ cup low-carb protein powder

¼ cup powdered erythritol

¼ cup shredded unsweetened coconut

¼ cup low-carb, sugar-free chocolate chips

½ teaspoon ground cinnamon

1 In a large bowl, mix almond butter and egg. Add in vanilla, protein powder, and erythritol.

2 Fold in coconut, chocolate chips, and cinnamon. Roll into 1" balls. Place balls into 6" round baking pan and put into the air fryer basket.

3 Adjust the temperature to 320°F and set the timer for 10 minutes.

4 Allow to cool completely. Store in an airtight container in the refrigerator up to 4 days.

PER SERVING

CALORIES: 224	FAT: 16.0 g
PROTEIN: 11.2 g	SODIUM: 40 mg
FIBER: 3.6 g	CARBOHYDRATES: 14.9 g
NET CARBOHYDRATES: 1.3 g	SUGAR: 1.3 g
SUGAR ALCOHOL: 10.0 g	

Cinnamon Sugar Pork Rinds

You might not have ever thought you'd be eating pork rinds for dessert, but this recipe is a true game changer. Pork rinds not only give you a protein boost, but they also give you a crunch that you just can't get from other low-carb snacks. The sweetness in this recipe will mask any meaty flavor, and your air fryer will make sure of that by baking the taste right in!

- **Hands-On Time: 5 minutes**
- **Cook Time: 5 minutes**

Serves 2

2 ounces pork rinds

2 tablespoons unsalted
    butter, melted

½ teaspoon ground cinnamon

¼ cup powdered erythritol

PORK RIND CEREAL?!

These sweet pork rinds also taste great if you're missing that cereal crunch! Crush them into bite-sized pieces and add a splash of unsweetened vanilla almond milk for a unique snack or quick breakfast.

1 In a large bowl, toss pork rinds and butter. Sprinkle with cinnamon and erythritol, then toss to evenly coat.

2 Place pork rinds into the air fryer basket.

3 Adjust the temperature to 400°F and set the timer for 5 minutes.

4 Serve immediately.

PER SERVING

CALORIES: 264

PROTEIN: 16.3 g

FIBER: 0.4 g

NET CARBOHYDRATES: 0.1 g

SUGAR ALCOHOL: 18.0 g

FAT: 20.8 g

SODIUM: 467 mg

CARBOHYDRATES: 18.5 g

SUGAR: 0.0 g

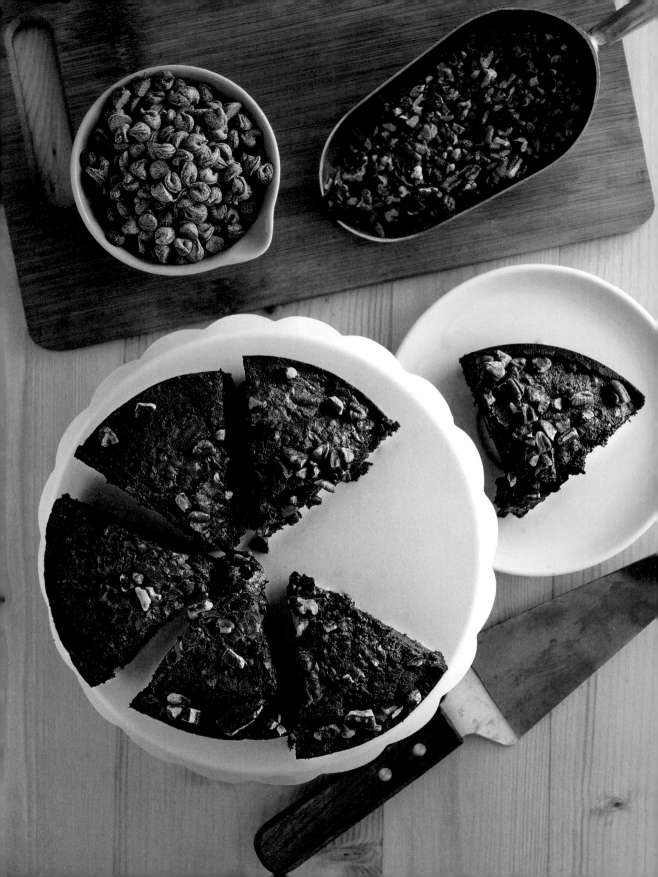

Pecan Brownies

These fudgy brownies are a dense and decadent dream. Finally, a chocolate-heavy, guilt-free dessert you can happily indulge in! And the pecans really hit the spot!

- **Hands-On Time: 10 minutes**
- **Cook Time: 20 minutes**

Serves 6

½ cup blanched finely ground almond flour

½ cup powdered erythritol

2 tablespoons unsweetened cocoa powder

½ teaspoon baking powder

¼ cup unsalted butter, softened

1 large egg

¼ cup chopped pecans

¼ cup low-carb, sugar-free chocolate chips

1 In a large bowl, mix almond flour, erythritol, cocoa powder, and baking powder. Stir in butter and egg.

2 Fold in pecans and chocolate chips. Scoop mixture into 6" round baking pan. Place pan into the air fryer basket.

3 Adjust the temperature to 300°F and set the timer for 20 minutes.

4 When fully cooked a toothpick inserted in center will come out clean. Allow 20 minutes to fully cool and firm up.

PER SERVING

CALORIES: 215	**FAT:** 18.9 g
PROTEIN: 4.2 g	**SODIUM:** 53 mg
FIBER: 2.8 g	**CARBOHYDRATES:** 21.8 g
NET CARBOHYDRATES: 2.3 g	**SUGAR:** 0.6 g
SUGAR ALCOHOL: 16.7 g	

Mini Cheesecake

This is the base of all keto-friendly cheesecakes you'll make in your air fryer. It's the classic vanilla cheesecake, but it can be customized so many different ways. From its crunchy walnut crust to its creamy center, this 15-minute cheesecake will quickly become a new favorite!

- **Hands-On Time: 10 minutes**
- **Cook Time: 15 minutes**

Serves 2

½ cup walnuts

2 tablespoons salted butter

2 tablespoons granular erythritol

4 ounces full-fat cream cheese, softened

1 large egg

½ teaspoon vanilla extract

⅛ cup powdered erythritol

LOW-CARB SWEETENERS

Erythritol is a low-glycemic sugar alcohol that can be used as a sweetener. There are other low-glycemic sweeteners, such as stevia, that can be used also, depending on your personal preference. Be aware of high-glycemic sugar alcohols, such as maltitol, which may spike your blood sugar.

1   Place walnuts, butter, and granular erythritol in a food processor. Pulse until ingredients stick together and a dough forms.

2   Press dough into 4" springform pan then place the pan into the air fryer basket.

3   Adjust the temperature to 400°F and set the timer for 5 minutes.

4   When timer beeps, remove the crust and let cool.

5   In a medium bowl, mix cream cheese with egg, vanilla extract, and powdered erythritol until smooth.

6   Spoon mixture on top of baked walnut crust and place into the air fryer basket.

7   Adjust the temperature to 300°F and set the timer for 10 minutes.

8   Once done, chill for 2 hours before serving.

PER SERVING

CALORIES: 531	FAT: 48.3 g
PROTEIN: 11.4 g	SODIUM: 333 mg
FIBER: 2.3 g	CARBOHYDRATES: 31.4 g
NET CARBOHYDRATES: 5.1 g	SUGAR: 2.9 g
SUGAR ALCOHOL: 24.0 g	

Chocolate Espresso Mini Cheesecake

This cheesecake definitely gives off major mocha vibes. Perfect for any sweet tooth out there that loves to enjoy a cup of coffee after dinner, this dessert is subtly rich and incredibly luscious.

- **Hands-On Time: 5 minutes**
- **Cook Time: 15 minutes**

Serves 2

½ cup walnuts

2 tablespoons salted butter

2 tablespoons granular erythritol

4 ounces full-fat cream cheese, softened

1 large egg

½ teaspoon vanilla extract

2 tablespoons powdered erythritol

2 teaspoons unsweetened cocoa powder

1 teaspoon espresso powder

1 Place walnuts, butter, and granular erythritol in a food processor. Pulse until ingredients stick together and a dough forms.

2 Press dough into 4" springform pan and place into the air fryer basket.

3 Adjust the temperature to 400°F and set the timer for 5 minutes.

4 When timer beeps, remove crust and let cool.

5 In a medium bowl, mix cream cheese with egg, vanilla extract, powdered erythritol, cocoa powder, and espresso powder until smooth.

6 Spoon mixture on top of baked walnut crust and place into the air fryer basket.

7 Adjust the temperature for 300°F and set the timer for 10 minutes.

8 Once done, chill for 2 hours before serving.

PER SERVING

CALORIES: 535	**FAT:** 48.4 g
PROTEIN: 11.6 g	**SODIUM:** 336 mg
FIBER: 7.2 g	**CARBOHYDRATES:** 37.1 g
NET CARBOHYDRATES: 5.9 g	**SUGAR:** 5.9 g
SUGAR ALCOHOL: 24.0 g	

Mini Chocolate Chip Pan Cookie

This quick dessert can bake before you even finish dinner! It's a very soft, chewy cookie thanks to the gelatin. To make this dessert even more special for a family treat, add a drizzle of low–carb chocolate syrup, your favorite roasted chopped nuts, and a dollop of sugar-free whipped cream!

- **Hands-On Time: 10 minutes**
- **Cook Time: 7 minutes**

Serves 4

½ cup blanched finely ground almond flour

¼ cup powdered erythritol

2 tablespoons unsalted butter, softened

1 large egg

½ teaspoon unflavored gelatin

½ teaspoon baking powder

½ teaspoon vanilla extract

2 tablespoons low-carb, sugar-free chocolate chips

1 In a large bowl, mix almond flour and erythritol. Stir in butter, egg, and gelatin until combined.

2 Stir in baking powder and vanilla and then fold in chocolate chips. Pour batter into 6″ round baking pan. Place pan into the air fryer basket.

3 Adjust the temperature to 300°F and set the timer for 7 minutes.

4 When fully cooked, the top will be golden brown and a toothpick inserted in center will come out clean. Let cool at least 10 minutes.

PER SERVING

CALORIES: 188	**FAT:** 15.7 g
PROTEIN: 5.6 g	**SODIUM:** 80 mg
FIBER: 2.0 g	**CARBOHYDRATES:** 16.8 g
NET CARBOHYDRATES: 2.3 g	**SUGAR:** 0.6 g
SUGAR ALCOHOL: 12.5 g	

Blackberry Crisp

You can enjoy certain fruits on a low-carb diet. Blackberries have one of the lowest glycemic indexes compared to other berries and are perfect to incorporate into a keto diet. This dessert is tart, fruity, and perfect for warm summer evenings! You can even top with a low–carb ice cream for extra decadence!

- **Hands-On Time: 5 minutes**
- **Cook Time: 15 minutes**

Serves 4

2 cups blackberries
⅓ cup powdered erythritol
2 tablespoons lemon juice
¼ teaspoon xanthan gum
1 cup Crunchy Granola
   (Chapter 2)

1 In a large bowl, toss blackberries, erythritol, lemon juice, and xanthan gum.

2 Pour into 6″ round baking dish and cover with foil. Place into the air fryer basket.

3 Adjust the temperature to 350°F and set the timer for 12 minutes.

4 When the timer beeps, remove the foil and stir.

5 Sprinkle granola over mixture and return to the air fryer basket.

6 Adjust the temperature to 320°F and set the timer for 3 minutes or until top is golden.

7 Serve warm.

PER SERVING

CALORIES: 496	**FAT:** 42.1 g
PROTEIN: 9.2 g	**SODIUM:** 5 mg
FIBER: 12.5 g	**CARBOHYDRATES:** 44.0 g
NET CARBOHYDRATES: 9./ g	**SUGAR:** 5.7 g
SUGAR ALCOHOL: 21.8 g	

Protein Powder Doughnut Holes

You can't forget about the doughnut holes...some would argue they're the best part! These poppable cake doughnut balls are great for breakfast or for dessert!

- **Hands-On Time: 25 minutes**
- **Cook Time: 6 minutes**

Yields 12 holes (2 per serving)

½ cup blanched finely ground almond flour

½ cup low-carb vanilla protein powder

½ cup granular erythritol

½ teaspoon baking powder

1 large egg

5 tablespoons unsalted butter, melted

½ teaspoon vanilla extract

WHAT'S UP WITH PROTEIN POWDER?

Protein powder is a very versatile ingredient. From fried chicken coating to baked goods, it can add volume while keeping carbs minimal. For desserts, flavored powder can really elevate a dish without adding extra carbs. Look for low-carb protein powders that use stevia, erythritol, or other low-glycemic sweeteners. You can also find unflavored protein powders to utilize in savory dishes.

1 Mix all ingredients in a large bowl. Place into the freezer for 20 minutes.

2 Wet your hands with water and roll the dough into twelve balls.

3 Cut a piece of parchment to fit your air fryer basket. Working in batches as necessary, place doughnut holes into the air fryer basket on top of parchment.

4 Adjust the temperature to 380°F and set the timer for 6 minutes.

5 Flip doughnut holes halfway through the cooking time.

6 Let cool completely before serving.

PER SERVING

CALORIES: 221	**FAT:** 14.3 g
PROTEIN: 19.8 g	**SODIUM:** 160 mg
FIBER: 1.7 g	**CARBOHYDRATES:** 23.2 g
NET CARBOHYDRATES: 1.5 g	**SUGAR:** 0.4 g
SUGAR ALCOHOL: 20.0 g	

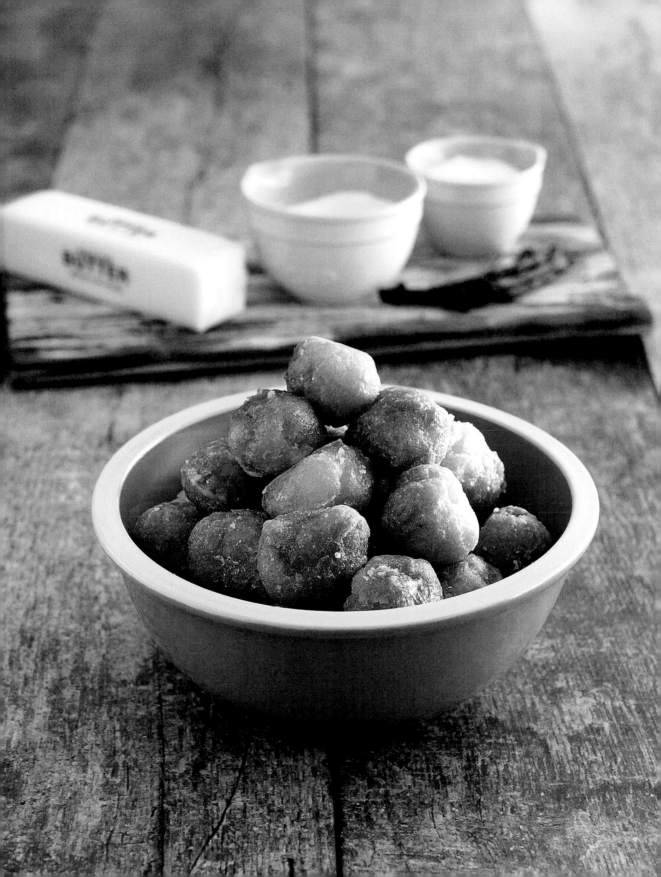

Layered Peanut Butter Cheesecake Brownies

This layered dessert is decadent, creamy, and perfect for a special occasion! Your guests won't even know it's low-carb. The rich chocolaty brownies make a great base for the fluffy peanut butter cheesecake layer. Add an extra drizzle of chocolate over the top for an extra special presentation.

- **Hands-On Time: 20 minutes**
- **Cook Time: 35 minutes**

Serves 6

½ cup blanched finely ground almond flour

1 cup powdered erythritol, divided

2 tablespoons unsweetened cocoa powder

½ teaspoon baking powder

¼ cup unsalted butter, softened

2 large eggs, divided

8 ounces full-fat cream cheese, softened

¼ cup heavy whipping cream

1 teaspoon vanilla extract

2 tablespoons no-sugar-added peanut butter

1 In a large bowl, mix almond flour, ½ cup erythritol, cocoa powder, and baking powder. Stir in butter and one egg.

2 Scoop mixture into 6" round baking pan. Place pan into the air fryer basket.

3 Adjust the temperature to 300°F and set the timer for 20 minutes.

4 When fully cooked a toothpick inserted in center will come out clean. Allow 20 minutes to fully cool and firm up.

5 In a large bowl, beat cream cheese, remaining ½ cup erythritol, heavy cream, vanilla, peanut butter, and remaining egg until fluffy.

6 Pour mixture over cooled brownies. Place pan back into the air fryer basket.

7 Adjust the temperature to 300°F and set the timer for 15 minutes.

8 Cheesecake will be slightly browned and mostly firm with a slight jiggle when done. Allow to cool, then refrigerate 2 hours before serving.

PER SERVING

CALORIES: 347	**FAT:** 30.9 g
PROTEIN: 8.3 g	**SODIUM:** 207 mg
FIBER: 2.0 g	**CARBOHYDRATES:** 29.8 g
NET CARBOHYDRATES: 3.8 g	**SUGAR:** 2.2 g
SUGAR ALCOHOL: 24.0 g	

Pumpkin Spice Pecans

These are a great addition to salads and desserts and your snack drawer as well! Pecans are a perfect fit for a ketogenic diet because they have high-fat, moderate-protein, and low-carb content. These pecans also taste great with a little cream cheese sandwiched between them as a treat!

- **Hands-On Time: 5 minutes**
- **Cook Time: 6 minutes**

Serves 4

1 cup whole pecans
¼ cup granular erythritol
1 large egg white
½ teaspoon ground cinnamon
½ teaspoon pumpkin pie spice
½ teaspoon vanilla extract

1 Toss all ingredients in a large bowl until pecans are coated. Place into the air fryer basket.

2 Adjust the temperature to 300°F and set the timer for 6 minutes.

3 Toss two to three times during cooking.

4 Allow to cool completely. Store in an airtight container up to 3 days.

PER SERVING

CALORIES: 178	FAT: 17.0 g
PROTEIN: 3.2 g	SODIUM: 13 mg
FIBER: 2.6 g	CARBOHYDRATES: 19.0 g
NET CARBOHYDRATES: 1.4 g	SUGAR: 1.1 g
SUGAR ALCOHOL: 15.0 g	

Coconut Flour Mug Cake

Coconut flour is a great substitute for almond flour in ketogenic baking. It has a sweeter taste and is more absorbent than almond flour, so you'll need only about a third as much when swapping it in. It's also the perfect trade when you're trying to avoid nut allergies!

- **Hands-On Time: 5 minutes**
- **Cook Time: 25 minutes**

Serves 1

1 large egg
2 tablespoons coconut flour
2 tablespoons heavy whipping cream
2 tablespoons granular erythritol
¼ teaspoon vanilla extract
¼ teaspoon baking powder

1 In a 4" ramekin, whisk egg, then add remaining ingredients. Stir until smooth. Place into the air fryer basket.

2 Adjust the temperature to 300°F and set the timer for 25 minutes. When done a toothpick should come out clean. Enjoy right out of the ramekin with a spoon. Serve warm.

PER SERVING

CALORIES: 237	FAT: 16.4 g
PROTEIN: 9.9 g	SODIUM: 213 mg
FIBER: 5.0 g	CARBOHYDRATES: 40.7 g
NET CARBOHYDRATES: 5.7 g	SUGAR: 4.2 g
SUGAR ALCOHOL: 30.0 g	

Pumpkin Cookie with Cream Cheese Frosting

This cookie is filled with the perfect flavors for fall. The soft spiced cookie complements the creamy frosting and makes a quick and slightly savory treat.

- **Hands-On Time: 10 minutes**
- **Cook Time: 7 minutes**

Serves 6

½ cup blanched finely ground almond flour

½ cup powdered erythritol, divided

2 tablespoons butter, softened

1 large egg

½ teaspoon unflavored gelatin

½ teaspoon baking powder

½ teaspoon vanilla extract

½ teaspoon pumpkin pie spice

2 tablespoons pure pumpkin purée

½ teaspoon ground cinnamon, divided

¼ cup low-carb, sugar-free chocolate chips

3 ounces full-fat cream cheese, softened

1 In a large bowl, mix almond flour and ¼ cup erythritol. Stir in butter, egg, and gelatin until combined.

2 Stir in baking powder, vanilla, pumpkin pie spice, pumpkin purée, and ¼ teaspoon cinnamon, then fold in chocolate chips.

3 Pour batter into 6" round baking pan. Place pan into the air fryer basket.

4 Adjust the temperature to 300°F and set the timer for 7 minutes.

5 When fully cooked, the top will be golden brown and a toothpick inserted in center will come out clean. Let cool at least 20 minutes.

6 To make the frosting: mix cream cheese, remaining ¼ teaspoon cinnamon, and remaining ¼ cup erythritol in a large bowl. Using an electric mixer, beat until it becomes fluffy. Spread onto the cooled cookie. Garnish with additional cinnamon if desired.

PER SERVING

CALORIES: 199	**FAT:** 16.2 g
PROTEIN: 4.8 g	**SODIUM:** 105 mg
FIBER: 1.9 g	**CARBOHYDRATES:** 21.5 g
NET CARBOHYDRATES: 2.9 g	**SUGAR:** 1.1 g
SUGAR ALCOHOL: 16.7 g	

Toasted Coconut Flakes

If you love a crunchy topping on your low-carb ice cream or yogurt, these flakes are perfect! They add a little sweetness and a big crunch to any meal and take just a few minutes to prepare! They're also delicious as a snack on the go. Store them in a hard container such as a small glass mason jar while you're on the go so they don't get crushed.

- **Hands-On Time: 5 minutes**
- **Cook Time: 3 minutes**

Serves 4

1 cup unsweetened coconut flakes
2 teaspoons coconut oil
¼ cup granular erythritol
⅛ teaspoon salt

LIGHT AND SWEET!

Coconut flakes are much larger than shredded coconut and make a great snacking chip. They're delicious by themselves but also taste great on top of low-carb ice cream or a keto-friendly cake. Make sure to check your labels to be positive they don't have any sneaky added sugars!

1 Toss coconut flakes and oil in a large bowl until coated. Sprinkle with erythritol and salt.

2 Place coconut flakes into the air fryer basket.

3 Adjust the temperature to 300°F and set the timer for 3 minutes.

4 Toss the flakes when 1 minute remains. Add an extra minute if you would like a more golden coconut flake.

5 Store in an airtight container up to 3 days.

PER SERVING

CALORIES: 165	**FAT:** 15.5 g
PROTEIN: 1.3 g	**SODIUM:** 76 mg
FIBER: 2.7 g	**CARBOHYDRATES:** 20.3 g
NET CARBOHYDRATES: 2.6 g	**SUGAR:** 0.5 g
SUGAR ALCOHOL: 15.0 g	

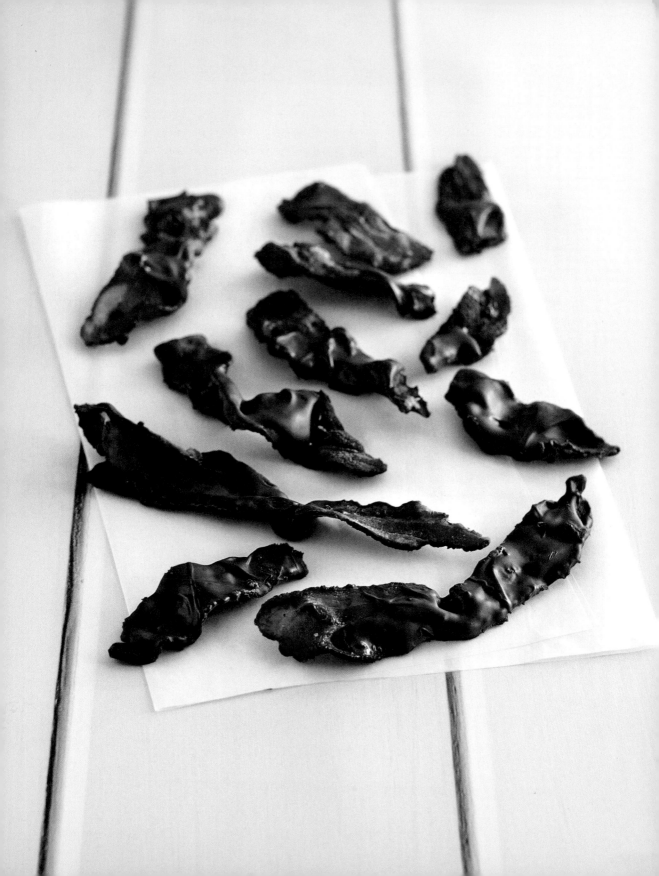

Chocolate-Covered Maple Bacon

Sweet and salty just go together. And this Chocolate-Covered Maple Bacon is an easy way to get in protein and fat while satisfying your sweet tooth! For added crunch, try sprinkling on some crushed almonds after you dip the bacon in chocolate!

- **Hands-On Time: 5 minutes**
- **Cook Time: 12 minutes**

Serves 2

8 slices sugar-free bacon

1 tablespoon granular erythritol

⅓ cup low-carb, sugar-free chocolate chips

1 teaspoon coconut oil

½ teaspoon maple extract

LOW-CARB CHOCOLATE

Low-carb chocolate can be hard to come by, but it's definitely out there! Lily's Sweets is a popular brand of stevia-sweetened chocolates that are available in bars and chocolate chips.

1 Place bacon into the air fryer basket and sprinkle with erythritol.

2 Adjust the temperature to 350°F and set the timer for 12 minutes.

3 Turn bacon halfway through the cooking time. Cook to desired doneness, checking at 9 minutes. (Smaller air fryers will cook much faster.)

4 When bacon is done, set aside to cool.

5 In a small microwave-safe bowl, place chocolate chips and coconut oil. Microwave for 30 seconds and stir. Add in maple extract.

6 Place bacon onto a sheet of parchment. Drizzle chocolate over bacon and place in refrigerator to cool and harden, about 5 minutes.

PER SERVING

CALORIES: 379	FAT: 25.9 g
PROTEIN: 15.3 g	SODIUM: 649 mg
FIBER: 2.7 g	CARBOHYDRATES: 31.8 g
NET CARBOHYDRATES: 3.0 g	SUGAR: 0.2 g
SUGAR ALCOHOL: 26.1 g	

Vanilla Pound Cake

This simple vanilla cake is a moist and delicious dessert that can also be used as a base for other cake flavors. Add fresh strawberries to the batter for a strawberry cake or even fresh lime juice for a citrus feel!

- **Hands-On Time: 10 minutes**
- **Cook Time: 25 minutes**

Serves 6

1 cup blanched finely ground almond flour
¼ cup salted butter, melted
½ cup granular erythritol
1 teaspoon vanilla extract
1 teaspoon baking powder
½ cup full-fat sour cream
1 ounce full-fat cream cheese, softened
2 large eggs

NUT ALLERGY?

To make any almond flour baked good nut-free, simply swap in coconut flour for ⅓ the amount of almond flour the recipe calls for. Coconut flour is very absorbent, so you need less of it in baking. The subtle hints of sweetness add a great flavor to desserts.

1. In a large bowl, mix almond flour, butter, and erythritol.

2. Add in vanilla, baking powder, sour cream, and cream cheese and mix until well combined. Add eggs and mix.

3. Pour batter into a 6″ round baking pan. Place pan into the air fryer basket.

4. Adjust the temperature to 300°F and set the timer for 25 minutes.

5. When the cake is done, a toothpick inserted in center will come out clean. The center should not feel wet. Allow it to cool completely, or the cake will crumble when moved.

PER SERVING

CALORIES: 253	**FAT:** 22.6 g
PROTEIN: 6.9 g	**SODIUM:** 191 mg
FIBER: 2.0 g	**CARBOHYDRATES:** 25.2 g
NET CARBOHYDRATES: 3.2 g	**SUGAR:** 1.5 g
SUGAR ALCOHOL: 20.0 g	

Chocolate Mayo Cake

You'll be in chocolate heaven with this simple yet decadent chocolate cake. It stays mouthwateringly moist in the middle, thanks to the mayonnaise, making this cake the perfect tool for conquering your chocolate cravings!

- **Hands-On Time: 10 minutes**
- **Cook Time: 25 minutes**

Serves 6

1 cup blanched finely ground almond flour

¼ cup salted butter, melted

½ cup plus 1 tablespoon granular erythritol

1 teaspoon vanilla extract

¼ cup full-fat mayonnaise

¼ cup unsweetened cocoa powder

2 large eggs

1 In a large bowl, mix all ingredients until smooth.

2 Pour batter into a 6″ round baking pan. Place into the air fryer basket.

3 Adjust the temperature to 300°F and set the timer for 25 minutes.

4 When done, a toothpick inserted in center will come out clean. Allow cake to cool completely, or it will crumble when moved.

PER SERVING

CALORIES: 270	FAT: 25.1 g
PROTEIN: 7.0 g	SODIUM: 143 mg
FIBER: 3.3 g	CARBOHYDRATES: 28.8 g
NET CARBOHYDRATES: 3.0 g	SUGAR: 0.9 g
SUGAR ALCOHOL: 22.5 g	

Raspberry Danish Bites

These bites are great for those who love shortbread cookies. The cookies themselves are fluffy and moist, and paired with the raspberry preserves they are the perfect snack. Feel free to use your favorite flavor of fruit preserves, just be sure to check the labels to make sure there are no added sugars or high-glycemic sweeteners.

- **Hands-On Time: 30 minutes**
- **Cook Time: 7 minutes**

Serves 10

1 cup blanched finely ground almond flour

1 teaspoon baking powder

3 tablespoons granular Swerve

2 ounces full-fat cream cheese, softened

1 large egg

10 teaspoons sugar-free raspberry preserves

ADD SOME ICE CREAM!

These bites taste great with some ice cream. To make an easy no-churn ice cream simply add 1 cup heavy whipping cream, ½ teaspoon vanilla extract, and ½ cup powdered erythritol to a large bowl and whisk until fluffy. Place in the freezer 1–2 hours until semi-firm.

1 Mix all ingredients except preserves in a large bowl until a wet dough forms.

2 Place the bowl in the freezer for 20 minutes until dough is cool and able to roll into a ball.

3 Roll dough into ten balls and press gently in the center of each ball. Place 1 teaspoon preserves in the center of each ball.

4 Cut a piece of parchment to fit your air fryer basket. Place each Danish bite on the parchment, pressing down gently to flatten the bottom.

5 Adjust the temperature to 400°F and set the timer for 7 minutes.

6 Allow to cool completely before moving, or they will crumble.

PER SERVING

CALORIES: 96		**FAT:** 7.7 g	
PROTEIN: 3.4 g		**SODIUM:** 76 mg	
FIBER: 1.3 g		**CARBOHYDRATES:** 9.8 g	
NET CARBOHYDRATES: 4.0 g		**SUGAR:** 2.4 g	
SUGAR ALCOHOL: 4.5 g			

Cream Cheese Danish

This Danish can double as a dessert or a sweet treat for breakfast! It's easy to make and pairs well with your favorite low-carb fruits. It tastes especially good alongside coffee or tea!

- **Hands-On Time: 20 minutes**
- **Cook Time: 15 minutes**

Serves 6

¾ cup blanched finely ground almond flour

1 cup shredded mozzarella cheese

5 ounces full-fat cream cheese, divided

2 large egg yolks

¾ cup powdered erythritol, divided

2 teaspoons vanilla extract, divided

1 In a large microwave-safe bowl, add almond flour, mozzarella, and 1 ounce cream cheese. Mix and then microwave for 1 minute.

2 Stir and add egg yolks to the bowl. Continue stirring until soft dough forms. Add ½ cup erythritol to dough and 1 teaspoon vanilla.

3 Cut a piece of parchment to fit your air fryer basket. Wet your hands with warm water and press out the dough into a ¼"-thick rectangle.

4 In a medium bowl, mix remaining cream cheese, erythritol, and vanilla. Place this cream cheese mixture on the right half of the dough rectangle. Fold over the left side of the dough and press to seal. Place into the air fryer basket.

5 Adjust the temperature to 330°F and set the timer for 15 minutes.

6 After 7 minutes, flip over the Danish.

7 When the timer beeps, remove the Danish from parchment and allow to completely cool before cutting.

PER SERVING

CALORIES: 185

PROTEIN: 7.4 g

FIBER: 0.5 g

NET CARBOHYDRATES: 2.3 g

SUGAR ALCOHOL: 18.0 g

FAT: 14.5 g

SODIUM: 205 mg

CARBOHYDRATES: 20.8 g

SUGAR: 1.3 g

Caramel Monkey Bread

This isn't your mama's monkey bread! Packed with protein and low on carbs, this caramel monkey bread is so delicious your non-keto friends will be asking for the recipe! Although erythritol doesn't caramelize in the same way sugar traditionally does, it still creates a flavorful and sticky alternative that will have you forgetting all about the sugar.

- **Hands-On Time: 15 minutes**
- **Cook Time: 12 minutes**

Serves 6 (2 pieces per serving)

½ cup blanched finely ground almond flour

½ cup low-carb vanilla protein powder

¾ cup granular erythritol, divided

½ teaspoon baking powder

8 tablespoons salted butter, melted and divided

1 ounce full-fat cream cheese, softened

1 large egg

¼ cup heavy whipping cream

½ teaspoon vanilla extract

1 In a large bowl, combine almond flour, protein powder, ½ cup erythritol, baking powder, 5 tablespoons butter, cream cheese, and egg. A soft, sticky dough will form.

2 Place the dough in the freezer for 20 minutes. It will be firm enough to roll into balls. Wet your hands with warm water and roll into twelve balls. Place the balls into a 6" round baking dish.

3 In a medium skillet over medium heat, melt remaining butter with remaining erythritol. Lower the heat and continue stirring until mixture turns golden, then add cream and vanilla. Remove from heat and allow it to thicken for a few minutes while you continue to stir.

4 While the mixture cools, place baking dish into the air fryer basket.

5 Adjust the temperature to 320°F and set the timer for 6 minutes.

6 When the timer beeps, flip the monkey bread over onto a plate and slide it back into the baking pan. Cook an additional 4 minutes until all the tops are brown.

7 Pour the caramel sauce over the monkey bread and cook an additional 2 minutes. Let cool completely before serving.

PER SERVING

CALORIES: 322	FAT: 24.5 g
PROTEIN: 20.4 g	SODIUM: 301 mg
FIBER: 1.7 g	CARBOHYDRATES: 33.7 g
NET CARBOHYDRATES: 2.0 g	SUGAR: 0.9 g
SUGAR ALCOHOL: 30.0 g	

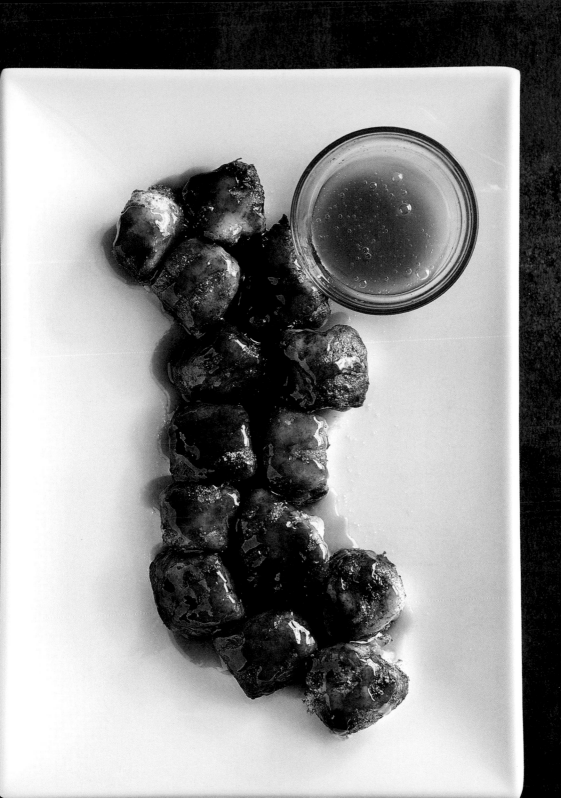

Cinnamon Cream Puffs

This recipe is perfect for Sunday brunch! The sweet dough is loaded with protein to keep you going while the inside has fragrant cinnamon to make this treat even more delicious! If you want a chocolate filling instead, simply add a tablespoon of cocoa powder to the filling!

- **Hands-On Time: 15 minutes**
- **Cook Time: 6 minutes**

Yields 8 puffs (1 per serving)

½ cup blanched finely ground almond flour

½ cup low-carb vanilla protein powder

½ cup granular erythritol

½ teaspoon baking powder

1 large egg

5 tablespoons unsalted butter, melted

2 ounces full-fat cream cheese

¼ cup powdered erythritol

¼ teaspoon ground cinnamon

2 tablespoons heavy whipping cream

½ teaspoon vanilla extract

1 Mix almond flour, protein powder, granular erythritol, baking powder, egg, and butter in a large bowl until a soft dough forms.

2 Place the dough in the freezer for 20 minutes. Wet your hands with water and roll the dough into eight balls.

3 Cut a piece of parchment to fit your air fryer basket. Working in batches as necessary, place the dough balls into the air fryer basket on top of parchment.

4 Adjust the temperature to 380°F and set the timer for 6 minutes.

5 Flip cream puffs halfway through the cooking time.

6 When the timer beeps, remove the puffs and allow to cool.

7 In a medium bowl, beat the cream cheese, powdered erythritol, cinnamon, cream, and vanilla until fluffy.

8 Place the mixture into a pastry bag or a storage bag with the end snipped. Cut a small hole in the bottom of each puff and fill with some of the cream mixture.

9 Store in an airtight container up to 2 days in the refrigerator.

PER SERVING

CALORIES: 178	**FAT:** 12.1 g
PROTEIN: 14.9 g	**SODIUM:** 121 mg
FIBER: 1.3 g	**CARBOHYDRATES:** 22.1 g
NET CARBOHYDRATES: 1.3 g	**SUGAR:** 0.4 g
SUGAR ALCOHOL: 19.5 g	

Pan Peanut Butter Cookies

Sometimes you just need a good peanut butter cookie. These four-ingredient treats can conquer your cravings in minutes! Thanks to the air fryer's small cooking chamber, you'll get an even, all around bake in no time for the perfect cookies!

- **Hands-On Time: 5 minutes**
- **Cook Time: 8 minutes**

Serves 8

1 cup no-sugar-added smooth peanut butter
⅓ cup granular erythritol
1 large egg
1 teaspoon vanilla extract

1 In a large bowl, mix all ingredients until smooth. Continue stirring for 2 additional minutes, and the mixture will begin to thicken.

2 Roll the mixture into eight balls and press gently down to flatten into 2″ round disks.

3 Cut a piece of parchment to fit your air fryer and place it into the basket. Place the cookies onto the parchment, working in batches as necessary.

4 Adjust the temperature to 320°F and set the timer for 8 minutes.

5 Flip the cookies at the 6-minute mark. Serve completely cooled.

PER SERVING

CALORIES: 210
PROTEIN: 8.8 g
FIBER: 2.0 g
NET CARBOHYDRATES: 2.1 g
SUGAR ALCOHOL: 10.0 g

FAT: 17.5 g
SODIUM: 8 mg
CARBOHYDRATES: 14.1 g
SUGAR: 1.1 g

Index